T5-ARD-889

# THE

# AYURVEDA  COOKBOOK

## Cooking  for Life

# The

# AyurVeda Cookbook

## Cooking for Life

American Edition

## LINDA BANCHEK

Illustrations by
Elaine Arnold

THE AYURVEDA COOKBOOK   Cooking For Life

Copyright 1989 by Linda Banchek
Printed in the United States of America.
All Rights Reserved.
No part of this book may be reproduced in any form or by any electronic or
mechanical means including information storage and retrieval systems without permission in writing from the publisher, except by a reviewer who may
quote brief passages in a review.

Published by Orchids & Herbs Press
503 W. Burlington, Box 1082, Fairfield, Iowa 52556

First Edition

LIBRARY OF CONGRESS CATALOGING IN PUBLICATION DATA
89-09206
Banchek, Linda
The AyurVeda Cookbook: Cooking for Life
Bibliography: p
1. Cookery — Health.   2. Ayurveda  I. Title

ISBN: 0-9623259-0-2

Dedicated to His Holiness Maharishi Mahesh Yogi in gratitude for his timely renewal of AyurVedic knowledge for the perfect health of our own and future generations.

Jai Guru Dev

This cookbook is going to be different from any other cookbook you've used. Oh, the foods, cooking styles, and recipes will seem familiar. Apple pie is, after all, apple pie. What makes this cookbook unique? When you use the ancient AyurVedic principles described here you will know just what effect your cooking is having on those who eat ... not in so many calories, grams of protein, and other intangibles, because each of us accumulates fat, burns calories, and digests protein in our own personal way. Instead, the AyurVeda Cookbook tells clearly and simply what you can expect when you eat, where you eat, depending on how and what you eat.

So now when you serve your best apple pie to those you love, you'll know what it's really doing for each of them. That's part of what AyurVedic cooking is about.

Please enjoy it!

# Table of Contents

## 1   About AyurVeda                                                   Page 1

This ancient "science of life" offers more than good cooking and good food. It brings practical knowledge to today's cooks and everyone who enjoys eating and living well. This chapter updates AyurVeda for contemporary health conscious Americans who either follow a vegetarian diet or simply want to maintain good health.

## 2   Cooking for Vata                                                 Page 19

What is Vata? How to identify the Vata body type with its special characteristics and prepare the best diet for those following a Vata- reducing diet. Vata menu planning and cooking tips, an ingredients chart, and the other information is presented, including a sample dinner menu with recipes, and a set of other main meal recipes especially good for Vata.

## 3   Cooking for Pitta                                                Page 41

What is Pitta? How to identify the Pitta body type and its special characteristics and prepare the best diet for balancing Pitta types. Present here are Pitta menu planning, cooking tips, seasonal considerations, staple items in Pitta's pantry, an ingredients chart, and all you need to follow a Pitta- reducing diet, including a sample dinner menu and a set of other main meal recipes especially good for Pitta and Pitta season.

## 4   Cooking for Kapha                                                Page 65

What is Kapha? How to identify the Kapha body type and its special characteristics and prepare the best diet for balancing Kapha, including seasonal considerations, menu planning, cooking tips, staples found in Kapha's pantry. There's an ingredients chart and all you need to follow a Kapha-reducing diet, including a sample dinner menu and a set of other main meal recipes especially good for Kapha types and Kapha season.

## 5   Planning Good Meals                                             Page 89

AyurVedic menu planning offers variety and balance, reflects the seasons, and relies especially on "common sense" in food selection. In this chapter you'll learn how to design you own recipes using foods that naturally combine well together, and how to plan well-balanced, delicious meals and more.

# Table of Contents

**6  Something For Everyone**                               *Page 105*

This chapter presents some universal Ayurvedic cooking principles, foods good for everyone to eat, and a few "basic little recipes" to keep handy.

**7  In the AyurVedic Kitchen**                             *Page 129*

How to be the best cook--an AyurVedic cook. Set up your own AyurVedic kitchen: proper food preparation, storage, utensils, and equipment.

**8  The AyurVeda Gourmet**                                 *Page 141*

Suggestions for entertaining with an international flavor. Sample menus to guide you in planning your own festivities. The menus and recipes include something from the French cuisine, a northern Italian dinner, elaborate dishes in the Indian style of cooking, and an American picnic.

**9  Special Diets**                                        *Page 187*

This chapter helps you follow a sensible diet, not fads, to lose weight, gives an eating program for new mothers with nourishing recipes, and offers general suggestions for healthy fasting.

**10  An AyurVeda Recipe Companion**                        *Page 215*

A collection of all the recipes that appear in this book and others.

**11  Questions and Answers about AyurVeda**                *Page 339*

Ayur-Veda physicians answer some commonly asked questions about diet.

*Appendices*                                               *Page 347*
 *All Dosha Ingredients Charts*                            *Page 349*
 *Glossary*                                                *Page 357*
 *Sources for Maharishi Ayur-Veda Information*             *Page 359*
 *Index*                                                   *Page 363*

*Acknowledgements*                                         *Page 367*

# Forward

Someone once said that irony is the point at which opposites meet and become one. Sometimes in researching and testing the foods for this book, irony became so tangible as to appear a separate ingredient in a recipe that read: "Take a pinch or more of irony and saute until transparent." The experience has given me insight into what it means for East to meet West. It was especially apparent during one research session when Dr. H. S. Kasture, a reknowned AyurVedic physician and professor (with mostly Indian food preferences) sat in a room on the plains of the American midwest, and using a most ancient system of food analysis, gave a rating to something that never appeared in the 5,000 year old Vedic literature--a scrumptious, typically American, chocolate custard pie.

On that day, after Dr. Kasture and two members of the AyurVeda research team had spent the morning intensely tasting and rating herbal teas, spices, and various fruits (after that much use, the taste buds usually lie back and refuse to register even one more sensation), and just as we were ready to quit, our cooks and research assistants arrived with the noontime meal for more tasting and evalution. On the menu: an Italian dinner, an American picnic, and some favorite desserts, including the wonderful chocolate pie. Everything looked and smelled so good that without hesitation we all began evaluating again with gusto!

That is how the research for this book was conducted. The cooks gave Dr. Kasture and his associate, Dr. Subhedar, servings of prepared foods and raw ingredients as well, and our AyurVeda experts would declare the specific qualities and effects these have on particular constitutions. They then recommended special considerations and menu alterations. In moments of doubt they consulted the appropriate Vedic texts, primarily the *Charaka Samhita*.

Sometimes they were asked to rate such things unfamilar to Indian tastes as parsley, French tarragon, thyme, or sage. When these were presented, the doctors' contemporary talents appeared. After a few rapid exchanges in Hindi and an occasional reference to a Sanskrit text, they would declare the qualities, tastes, and effects of each herb. I recorded this unusual application of the science of AyurVeda in an analysis of hundreds of ingredients and some popular recipes found in the contemporary Western vegetarian diet. And that is what has been collected in this book.

It is with sincere gratitude and a deep regard that I acknowledge my indebtedness to these brilliant AyurVedic physicians and scientists, Dr. Haridas Shridar Kasture and Dr. Pramod Dattatrya Subhedar, for putting into practice their firm belief that AyurVeda is a necessary part of modern life, Eastern and Western; and that the basic principles of this ancient science

can be lived by everyone. And I would especially like to thank His Holiness
Maharishi Mahesh Yogi for updating the knowledge from these and other
AyurVedic doctors and making it useful for us today.


Linda Banchek
Fairfield, Iowa

# Chapter 1

# About AyurVeda

## Using Ancient Knowledge Today

*AYURVEDA - From the ancient Sanskrit: Ayu* - life and *veda* - knowledge. Ayur-Veda includes all of life: consciousness, physiology, behavior, and environment. By following simple AyurVedic diet, good health and a comfortable sense of well-being naturally result. Although it originated in India more than 5,000 years ago, AyurVeda's concepts are as practical for us today as in ages past.

## AyurVedic Food

AyurVedic food is not exotic or unusual - unless you want it to be. It simply consists of any delicious food, properly cooked, with full knowledge of its effects on the health and satisfaction of the eater. Just because AyurVeda originated in India does not mean you can only eat Indian food to be healthy. For Americans, AyurVeda includes all the kinds of foods we usually enjoy in contemporary American cooking. To become an AyurVedic cook might only be a matter of adjusting some favorite recipes by increasing or decreasing certain seasonings and other ingredients to suit individual needs at particular times of the year. AyurVeda works everywhere. No matter the country, the same principles apply.

## Enjoyment and Health

By following AyurVedic principles when cooking and eating we become more aware of subtle nuances in the tastes and textures of what we are eating. With more attention to these finer aspects of our food, we grow in enjoyment of the whole process of eating.

*One should not make radical changes in dietary habits. It is enough if one changes gradually.*

-Maharishi Mahesh Yogi

3

# 1 The AyurVeda Cookbook

When we begin following AyurVedic dietary practices "grabbing a bite to eat" somehow loses its appeal. Every meal becomes an occasion for celebration and enjoyment. The first principle of the science of life is enjoyment.

## Balance and the Doshas

Recognizing the vital connection between a balanced diet and perfect health, AyurVeda provides a thorough understanding of nutrition useful for all constitutional types. Our bodies are made of the same essential elements found everywhere in nature: air and space, fire, water, and earth. According to AyurVeda, each person is naturally an identifiable constitutional type called VATA, PITTA, or KAPHA, or sometimes a combination of two or all three. Vata is most like air and space, Pitta like water and fire, and Kapha earth and water. When these elements are out of balance they are called *doshas*. By maintaining balance of the three doshas we enjoy good health. When the balance of these three essential elements is disturbed, illness results.

*Balance of doshas means that life is not allowed to go out of the field of wholeness. This is perfect health.*

- Richard Averbach, M.D

## To Maintain Balance

The key to maintaining good constitutional balance is to eat more of the foods that pacify a dominant dosha and less of foods that aggravate it. This does not mean eliminating all foods with certain qualities or tastes that don't appear on your list of dosha-specific foods; that would be done only on the advice of a qualified Maharishi Ayur-Vedic physician ( See Appendex). For instance, the salty taste increases both Pitta and Kapha doshas. To pacify these dominant doshas Pitta and Kapha types would generally reduce salt somewhat. But a reduced salt diet is *not* a salt-free diet. Some small amount of the salty taste is necessary at each main meal for Pitta and Kapha, but not very much.

## What is Your Body Type?

Right now you might want to identify your body type or constitution according to AyurVeda. This simple chart gives a general idea of the three body types.

| Vata Characteristics | Pitta Characteristics | Kapha Characteristics |
|---|---|---|
| • light, thinner build | • moderate build | • solid, heavier build |
| • performs activity quickly | • performs activity with medium speed | • slow, methodical activity |
| • tendency to dry skin | • tendency toward red complexion and hair, moles and freckles | • smooth, oily skin,hair is plentiful, tends to be darker |
| • irregular hunger and digestion, tendency toward constipation | • sharp hunger and digestion, can't skip meals, prefers cold food and drink | • slow digestion and mild hunger |
| • quick to grasp new information, also quick to forget | • medium time to grasp new information | • slow to grasp new information, slow to forget |
| • tendency to worry | • tendency toward irritability and temper | • tranquil, steady nature, slow to become excited or irritated |
| • often light and interrupted sleep | • enterprising and sharp character, good speakers | • sleep is heavy and long |
| • aversion to cold weather | • aversion to hot weather | • greater strength and endurance |

# 1 The AyurVeda Cookbook

## Similarities and Differences and the Universe

There are two principles in AyurVeda known as *Samanya* (similarities) and *Vishesha* (differences) or "Alikes" and "Unalikes." It explains how the body interacts with the world around it. And how the contents of the entire universe affect the body. AyurVeda sees the human body as a miniature of the universe. Anything, any element or law of nature, found in the universe can be found in a human body. This broad point of view is the basis for planning an individual's diet to maintain a balance between the inner workings of the body and changes in the environment.

Briefly, the rule is that any substance taken from outside of the body which is similar to something within the body will cause that within the body to increase. Likewise, anything taken from outside the body which is different from something within the body will cause that within the body to decrease. This is why the taste and qualities of foods most like one's body type increase that type. Like goes with like. So oily and cold, heavy, slow, smooth, sweet things that are like Kapha, anywhere in the environment, increase Kapha. Hot, salty, spicy, light, dry food increases active, fiery Pitta because they are most like Pitta. And all cold, dry, windy, light, bitter things are associated with Vata.

*Everything found in the universe is found in the human body. We take items from the universe, maintain them for a while, then release them.*

-Dr. H.S. Kasture

## AyurVedic Cooking and Eating

Whether discussing cooking or eating AyurVedic dieticians and physicians emphasize nourishment and enjoyment. They are less concerned with the relatively "new" concepts of caloric content, vitamins, minerals, fats, proteins, and carbohydrates than they are with proper digestion and the particular balance of food tastes and qualities that each person enjoys at each meal. This concept of the subtle effect of food taste and quality on nutrition, as well as enjoyment while eating and a good appetite, is the heart of AyurVedic nutrition. When you follow a properly designed AyurVedic diet all those nutrients currently listed as necessary for good health are naturally available.

AyurVeda takes into account effects of everything on an individual and gives advice about what and how to eat in order to stay healthy and avoid future illnesses. For most people who follow AyurVeda, cooking and eating will not necessitate any major dietary changes, but an adjustment of some eating habits may naturally occur as you become more aware of how tastes and textures, and even times of day and changing weather conditions, make differences in your state of health.

## Good Digestion and Good Health

Unless you are able to properly digest and assimilate what you eat, any nutritional information printed on food packages showing the amounts of protein, fats, and so forth per average serving is of little use to you. In AyurVeda, the main concern is that your digestive power, called *agni*, is working properly. If it is not, then even eating the freshest and most highly nutritious foods will be of uncertain use to us because they cannot be well assimilated by the body.

*Maintain your digestive power and eat.*
*Food is like fuel to the fire.*

- Dr. Subhedar

A strong appetite is a healthy sign of strong agni. But no matter how refined the food, how careful the preparation, and how beautiful the setting for dining, if digestion is not efficient nutrition will be poor. If the eater takes care of nutrition at its source — that is, by maintaining agni, the digestive fire — then good health will result.

## Ayurvedic Eating: A Refined Pleasure

AyurVeda applies a far more subtle understanding of the sensory perception of eating than most of us are accustomed to. As you read this book some food qualities or tastes such as salty and oily are obvious, but other descriptions are more refined. Until you become more experienced in identifying these, the Charts of Ingredients in the back of the book might be helpful.

## Food Tastes and Qualities

Properly balanced meals incorporate a variety of tastes and food qualities into every main meal. Of the many tastes and qualities that food ingredients can have, the six major ones used in this book are: SWEET, SALTY, SOUR, PUNGENT, ASTRINGENT, AND BITTER; HOT, COLD, DRY, OILY, HEAVY, AND LIGHT. In AyurVeda every taste and quality has a specific and known effect on the digestion. The chapters in this book devoted to diet for the particular body types of Vata, Pitta or Kapha list those foods best for balancing individual diet. And as a general reference the Charts of Ingredients list according to tastes, quality, and effects on each body type many commonly eaten fruits, vegetables, spices, herbs, beverages, grains, and other foods for a healthy diet.

# The Basic Food Tastes

Sweet • Salty • Sour • Astringent • Pungent • Bitter

## Flavor and Taste

First, it is important to note the difference in meaning between "flavor" and "taste." The concept of *taste* in AyurVeda is a general way to classify food groups according to their effects during the digestive process. Many flavors may be included in each taste. The distinct flavor of a food within the taste catagory makes it unique. *Flavor* is what makes eating so interesting. For example, there are many foods with a pungent or spicy taste, but they do not all have a "hot" or "spicy" flavor. Black pepper, basil, and saffron have the pungent taste. Each one's flavor is very different from the other. And the spicy or pungent effect of that taste is not necessarily on the tongue or palate. Saffron is a heating herb whose "taste" effect is a kind of secondary reaction in the stomach rather than in the mouth. On the palate it has a rather bland, sweet flavor.

## Examples of the Six Basic Tastes

### Sweet

When we think of a sweet taste, sugar or honey come to mind. But the sweet taste is not just sugar. Many foods such as rice, wheat, most fruits, some nuts, butter, milk, a few herbs and spices, and many vegetables have what Ayur-Veda considers a sweet taste. By briefly scanning the Ingredients Charts it is possible to find a variety of sweet foods, many in combination with other tastes, that may surprise you. These are just a few: artichokes, beets, cucumbers, oranges, persimmons, and squash. The sweet taste may be produced in the mouth or the stomach.

### Salty

If you want to add the salty taste to the diet you can use table salt.or such condiments as soy sauce, olives, pickles. Many processed foods taste salty. It is best to read the labels on packaged foods to find out how much salt, sugar, and other ingredients are being added to the product before packaging. This is especially true for breakfast cereals which contain much more than just wheat, oats, or other grains

### Sour

Some of the obvious foods with a sour taste are yogurt, cheese, grapefruit, and dill pickles. Some others are tomatoes, rosehips, green apples, rye bread, and peanuts. The sour taste in foods is experienced as sour in the mouth and during digestion. Sour dairy products take five or six hours to fully digest and should be eaten at the main meal of the day rather than in the evening or too close to bedtime.

### Pungent

Chili peppers and radishes are pungent. So are peppermint, cinnamon, parsley, sage, basil and thyme. Some pungent tastes are easy to identify at first bite. Others have their spicy effect later in digestion. For most people, using a small amount of pungent spices will make enough of this taste.. This is especially true in the summertime and for Pitta types.

### Astringent

The astringent taste is rather drying and "puckery." Vinegar is astringent. So are beans, lentils, chocolate, tumeric, rosemary, celery leaves, peas, apples, barley, corn, and olive oil. If this taste is not immediately noticeable in the mouth, it has its effect later in the digestive process.

### Bitter

The bitter taste is obvious with the first bite. It only varies in strength. Horseradish leaves and dandelion greens are two bitter and tonic herbs of spring. Chocolate, honey, walnuts, lettuce, and Swiss chard provide some bitterness to the diet as well.

# 1 *The AyurVeda Cookbook*

## The Qualities of Ingredients

In determining the quality of cooking ingredients, AyurVeda considers their internal effects as well as their textures, serving temperatures, or other obvious sensory characteristics. For instance, the qualities of hot or cold do not necessarily mean temperature in degrees of Fahrenheit, but their internal heating or cooling effects during digestion. So when we read that a steaming bowl of rice is "cold," it is not cold to the touch but inside the digestive system. Just as saffron is not "hot" until it arrives in the stomach, a food feels hot only in the mouth such as, a radish, or hot in the mouth and stomach like pungent chili peppers.

It's not necessary to remember where the quality occurs; just know that these qualities — hot, cold, heavy, light, dry and oily — may have their effect at more subtle levels of digestion. So when a particular food is listed here with a quality not immediately apparent, you'll know that it refers to its subtle AyurVedic effect. A few additional qualities, such as smooth, sharp, and so forth, are mentioned in the Ingredients Charts.

## The Basic Food Qualities

Light • Heavy • Dry • Oily • Hot • Cold

## Examples of the Six Basic Qualities

### LIGHT

Cereals, rice cakes, apples, celery, spinach, and other greens are light,. as are some ingredients that have been heated by boiling or quick frying in very little oil. Any ingredient with a light quality that takes less time to digest is a "food of choice" for Kapha types and those people who want to lose weight.

### HEAVY

Most high-protein food that is nourishing for all body tissues has a heavy quality. Those who do not need to reduce weight, including most Pitta and Vata types, should include heavy foods more than light ones in their diets. Some heavy foods are milk, potatoes, peaches, avocados, cucumbers, sugar, breads and wheat products, nuts, meat, tofu, and beans. The heavy quality may not be apparent until after eating, as a secondary part of digestion.

10

DRY

Many grains, spices, and vegetables are dry in quality. Broccoli, cabbage, eggplant, spinach, yams, barley, oats, cayenne and other peppers, nutmeg, ginger, and vinegar are dry. Dry and light qualities often seem to be found together. These are good for Kapha types and those reducing weight.

OILY

An oily quality is more than just an oily feel to the touch. It is unctuous—that is, internally lubricating. This is an important quality for those with dry skin or Pitta and Vata types, and an important dietary consideration in winter when the air is dry. Although cooking oils and ghee are obviously oily during eating, other foods provide the necessary unctuous quality later in digestion. Some of these are milk, nuts, coriander, lentils, asparagus, carrots, oats, and rice. Oily and heavy food qualities are often found in combination in "body building" foods.

*Unctuous Food*
*Provokes subtle digestive power*
*Digests quickly*
*Moves Vata downward*
*Increases physical strength*
*Improves the senses*
*Brings out full brightness of complexion*
- Charaka Samhita

HOT

Hot food does not necessarily mean pungent, spicy food or food right off the stove. The hot quality in food is usually found during the digestive process, rather than by touch. Heat is important for proper digestion, and the foods that are hot in quality are best for Vata and Kapha types who have less internal heat for good digestion. Some hot foods are corn, beans and lentils, seafood, turmeric, fenugreek, mustard seeds, asafoetida (hing), cloves, yogurt, and carrots.

COLD

In the same way, foods with a cold quality are often experienced as cold after tasting them. Some obviously cold foods are ice cream, cheese and milk, grapes, and other juicy fruits. Other cold foods include sugar, rice, wheat, lentils, artichokes, cucumbers, and zucchini.

## Good Digestion: Agni and the Three Doshas

Now that we know the basic tastes and qualities that make a balanced meal, we will consider the second most important requirement for proper nutrition: a good digestive fire or *agni* (pronounced AGH-nee).

*When one sits to eat*
*Food is the fuel*
*Digestion is the fire*
*This is yagya.*

-Dr. H.S. Kasture

Each of the three doshas has its own metabolic rate and its own degree of agni. Pitta, like the element of fire, has the most agni. People with Pitta constitutions have the best digestion. In fact, when they are hungry it is their digestive fire that makes them seem ravenous. And too much hot, dry, or pungent food can irritate fiery Pitta. Kapha is slow and some-times unsteady in digestion. And Vata often needs help igniting agni. Good appetizers are usually necessary for Vata and Kapha types to enjoy eating.

## Appetizers

What makes a good appetizer? Something with zip... something a little pungent, or warm, sweet, and unctuous or a combination of these. Serve just enough of an appetizer to spark digestion, not satisfy it. It can be as simple as a sweet pickle or gherkin, or a small amount of warm rice and ghee, or a relish of chopped fresh ginger, lemon juice, and salt. Even a pinch of ground ginger placed under the tongue just before eating will start the digestive fire and bring enjoyment to the whole meal.

## Eating Everything: A Balanced Diet

A balanced diet for anyone without specific health problems means eating some amount of all the tastes, qualities, and catagories (gunas) daily— even some of those things that increase a dominant dosha. For instance, people with dominant Kapha body types would not avoid all Kapha-increasing foods because many of these are considered "body builders" and maintainers of strength. Kapha metabolism is so efficient in turning body building foods into weight that those following a Kapha-reducing diet do not need large amounts of heavy, sweet, high protein, oily foods.  A balanced Kapha diet would include small amounts of Kapha-increasing foods and much larger portions of Kapha-decreasing foods.

The same idea of proportional balance applies for Pitta and Vata types. In the following chart you can see how different tastes and food qualities influence each body type either by increasing (+) or decreasing (-) it.

# Food Tastes

|            | VATA | PITTA | KAPHA |
|------------|------|-------|-------|
| Sweet      | -    | -     | +     |
| Sour       | -    | +     | +     |
| Salty      | -    | +     | +     |
| Pungent    | +    | +     | -     |
| Bitter     | +    | -     | -     |
| Astringent | +    | -     | -     |

(+) increases or aggravates  and  ( - ) decreases or calms.

## Food Qualities

|        | VATA | PITTA | KAPHA |
|--------|:----:|:-----:|:-----:|
| Heavy  | -    | -     | +     |
| Light  | +    | -     | -     |
| Dry    | +    | +     | -     |
| Oily   | -    | -     | +     |
| Hot    | -    | +     | -     |
| Cold   | +    | -     | +     |

## Satisfaction: Sign of a Balanced Diet

One practical test of good AyurVedic food comes with a welcome sense of comfort and well-being after eating. It is neither a feeling of being very full or hungry. Feelings of dissatisfaction or indigestion after eating a main meal can come from lack of balance in the ingredients used, from poor cooking techniques, eating too fast, or too much. Some people overeat as a habit, or they eat meals that have little satisfaction built into them. Some meals will satisfy one person and not another. Satisfying meals depend on whether the predominant tastes and qualities in the meal are good for that person and if the meal has been prepared with the cook's full attention.

## Breakfast: An Example

In AyurVeda breakfast is considered a light meal or nourishing snack to be eaten only if hungry. It is never a main meal. A typical American breakfast may include cereal with milk or cream, toast with butter, orange juice, tea or coffee. This is considered a light meal and both Pitta and Vata can start the day this way. But, with the exception of the tea and coffee, everything else increases Kapha. At first Kapha might feel "full," but since the food lacks balance in the tastes and qualities best for Kapha, it is not really satisfying. As a result, after a short time Kapha will want to snack. In the American tradition of the coffee break Kapha might have a mid-morning pastry and more coffee or tea. Again Kapha increasing and not satisfying. And snacking so frequently weakens agni for the main meal at noon. A good breakfast for Kapha is warm tea or coffee and something light and dry, such as rice cakes or a slice of cornbread, eaten plain or spread with a little ghee or nut butter.

## Digestion

AyurVeda encourages eating practices that maintain good digestive power. Indigestion is the result of eating too much heavy food that cannot be assimilated properly. Sometimes overeating is simply a habit of anticipating that we might have to miss a meal and so overfill the stomach to avoid hunger later. Overeating gives pressure to the heart causing discomfort, heartburn, gas, and a toxic substance called ama. Ama comes from improperly digested food, or food that passes "immaturely" through the digestive system and does not allow the plasma and body tissues to be formed on schedule. It is the source of many diseases.

Other causes of improper digestion are eating when angry or otherwise upset; eating sour dairy foods late in the evening, that is, too close to bedtime, thus slowing the digestive process before its conclusion; and frequent snacking or eating when the stomach is still digesting the previous meal. Waiting three to six hours between meals with no snacking, except perhaps to drink a glass of water, juice, tea, or milk in between, is considered ideal.

*Wisdom is knowing the difference between habitual demands made by the mind and the simple demands of the body.*
- Dr. H.S. Kasture

## Eat The Right Amount

A simple AyurVedic rule is always eat the proper quantity. The wisdom lies in knowing how much is enough. Filling the stomach to two-thirds capacity is the maximum for the best digestive activity . Too much food produces a feeling of fullness and heaviness or lethargy after eating. With too little food agni begins burning body tissues for fuel, thus causing loss of weight. But if we eat just a little less than what makes us feel full, then agni will remain strong. Overburdened agni becomes weak and disordered and cannot perform adequately. To give the digestive system a rest, AyurVeda recommends regular fasting for anyone who is not seriously ill, anemic, weak, pregnant, or nursing, and with a physician's approval.

# 1 The AyurVeda Cookbook

## Diet and the Environment

Dietary considerations in AyurVeda are based on the time of day when eating, the weather or seasons, and even the climate where we live and where the food is grown.

The time of eating is important. Breakfast, if eaten at all, should be taken as a light, easily-digested meal very early in the morning. The biggest meal of the day should be around noontime, that is, when agni is strongest in the environment. This is an example of the similarity between one's internal digestive fire and the external fire of the sun. It is thought that the digestive glands begin to secrete around 12:30 PM. When we eat food near that time the digestive enzymes will be used most efficiently . Invite guests to lunch for a spectacular feast that everyone can enjoy. A lighter evening meal is best eaten between 6:00 PM and 8:00 PM. If a heavy meal is eaten in the evening there is not enough time for it to fully digest before bedtime. Although a light meal only needs two or three hours to digest, it is good to allow five to six hours after eating a full meal for the stomach to empty before eating again.

*The ancient AyurVedic physicians noted that conditions are best for proper digestion while sunlight is greatest.*

In the summer eat fewer heavy, high protein foods than during the colder days of spring and winter. These foods are harder to digest and assimilate, and during the hot summer months one's internal agni is overpowered by the heat found in the environment..

## The Body: the Environment

Common sense dictates that you eat when you are hungry and not just when the clock says it is dinnertime. Sometimes you might really crave some taste or particular food that you know is contrary to your needs. But you want it! This is a good, healthy sign that a certain element is low or lacking in your body's chemistry. The longing for a certain taste or quality comes from the very cells of your body that have a need to be nourished in a specific way. The body hints at what it wants to eat. It is the mind that creates incorrect eating habits. Food selection is one way the body demonstrates its wisdom to maintain balance.

*The desire to eat arises from the level of the cell. It comes from the ultimate desire for balance.*

- Stuart Rothenberg. M.D

## Enjoy What You Eat

Ayurveda's advice is always to eat well of fresh, deliciously prepared food that pleases you. When you feel an urge to eat something that you know is not in your best interest, by all means enjoy a little of it. You don't have to deprive yourself, or wait until the weather changes or the season, or until you've had a chance to consult a certain food chart.

AyurVeda is like a tender-hearted mother who never likes to say, "No." Instead she says, "Just taste a little."

Except for a few things that really shouldn't be eaten at certain times — such as yogurt, cheese, and sour cream late at night, or such unhealthy combinations as milk and seafood, or equal parts of honey and ghee, foods cooked with honey, and carbonated drinks with food — you should eat what pleases you. Eat just enough to satisfy your desire, then let it go.

## Climate

The climate in which food is grown and where one lives also affects the diet when following the principle of similarities and differences. Foods grown in dry areas and deserts tend to have light qualities, while those grown in moist, warm areas have heavy qualities. When living in humid or moist climates, it is best to eat more of hot, dry, and light foods. And when living in dry areas add many cooler and more oily, heavy foods to your diet.

# 1 The AyurVeda Cookbook

## Common Sense: The Empty Bag

Dr. Kasture tells a story of an AyurVedic physician who takes his shopping bag and goes to the market to buy food for dinner. All the beautiful fresh foods are displayed there in abundance.

First the man begins filling his bag with lots of little pink skinned potatoes. "Uh, oh, these will increase my Vata," he says, and puts them back.

He then selects some luscious, red tomatoes, but just as he fills his bag, he remembers that tomatoes increase Pitta. So he returns them.

At the fruit stand the man picks an inviting pineapple, a bunch of bananas, and a few oranges. Then he thinks to himself, "All these fruits increase my Kapha, I'll have to put them back."

And he walks home to dinner with an empty bag.

Be good eater, follow common sense, and eat from a full bag.

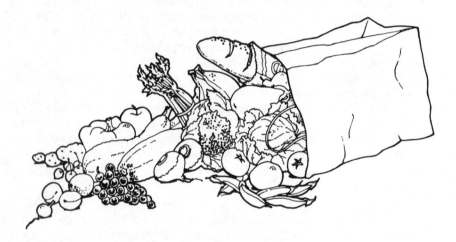

*Chapter 2*

# *Cooking for Vata*

## What is Vata?

By nature everyone is one of the three essential types: Vata, Pitta, Kapha, or perhaps a combination of these three. Vata is most like air and space. It is dry, cold, windy, and lightweight. Your nature is most like Vata if many of the characteristics in this list best descibe you.

# Vata Characteristics

| Balanced | Out of Balance |
| --- | --- |
| Vivacious | Restless |
| Joyful, serene | Nervous, or flighty |
| Alert, quick learner | Forgetful, spacey |
| Confident | Anxious, worried |
| Light but sound sleep | Difficulty sleeping |
| Moves lightly, gracefully | Body stiff and slow |
| Smooth skin, regular bowels | Dry skin, constipated |

## The Best Diet For Vata

Following a Vata-balancing diet is one way AyurVeda suggests to maintain health. If Vata is out of balance follow a good Vata-reducing diet and visit an AyurVeda physician, too.

Vata types and any combinations that include the element of Vata, such as Vata-Kapha, Vata-Pitta, and Vata-Pitta-Kapha, should follow a Vata-balancing diet during winter and very early spring or whenever the cold, dry, windy weather that is most disturbing to Vata types prevails in your locale. Those with Vata nature only follow a Vata-balancing diet all year round.

# General Vata Diet

## Favor

- Warm, Delicious Food, and Drink
- Tastes: Sweet, Sour, and Salty
- Qualities: Heavy, Hot, and Oily
- Small To Moderate Amounts Of Food
- Eat Frequently - Every Four To Five Hours
- Enjoy Rich Foods

## Reduce

- Cold Food
- Chilled Drinks
- Weight-Reducing Food
- Tastes: Bitter, Astringent, Pungent
- Qualities: Cold, Dry, Light
- Very Heavy and Infrequent Meals

## Tastes and Qualities Best for Vata

Certain food tastes and qualities are best for Vata types. For a balanced meal serve all six tastes and six qualties but eat most of those foods that reduce Vata.

# Best Food Tastes for Vata

- Sweet • Sour • Salty •

## Menu Planning for Vata

Warm, sweet, sour, salty, slightly pungent foods good for body building and strength are best for people with Vata chacteristics. Vata, most like the element of wind or air, is bothered in windy, dry , or cold weather. During these days when agni, that fiery element, is neither very active in the environment nor in Vata's digestive system, people with this constitution find it difficult to feel warm inside or to digest food effectively. They should particularly avoid raw or undercooked vegetables, light snacks, cold drinks, and carbonated beverages.

Soups provide a warm, appetizing start to a meal for everyone — especially Vata types. They should be served frequently, even at every main meal, during Vata season. A steaming bowl of bouillon or a tasty, thin vegetable soup appears as a regular feature in Vata's menu plan, even in the summer. Good nourishing soups do not necessarily have to be thick or heavy.

# Best Food Qualities for Vata

• Heavy • Hot • Oily •

The most useful menus for Vata begin with several selections that are delicious and stimulating to the appetite, and then continue with one nourishing main dish with heavy, oily qualities served during the middle of the meal. If a thick soup is to be served, it should be preceded by a good appetizer; otherwise, it would be better eaten as the main part of a light meal with bread and a salad. Serving a heavy soup as an appetizer to Vata has a good chance of shutting down the digestive fire and ending Vata's interest early in the meal.

## Balance

If someone following a Vata-balancing diet eats many substantial, warm, rich, nourishing foods good things naturally happen. He or she thrives and does not feel hungry right after eating, digestion works efficiently, skin and hair look healthy, and physical stamina remains constant. As long as a Vata type eats in a balanced way at lunch and dinner, without between meal snacking, he will maintain good digestive power and the ability to get the most nutrients from his food.

*A proper diet*
*purifies the physiology,*
*gives strength and energy,*
*promotes health and clear thinking,*
*maintains life*

-The Upanishads

It is especially after eating meals made up of undercooked or light, dry foods that Vata types remain hungry and feel dissatisfied and uncomfortable. The rice cakes that satisfy Kapha are too light for Vata. And vegetables that are briefly steamed but still crunchy are fine for Pitta, but are difficult for Vata to digest.

## Satisfaction

It is an important point to remember in planning an AyurVedic menu to include all six tastes and six qualities in both lunch and dinner. A healthy meal will consist of mostly sweet, salty, sour, heavy, oily, and hot ingredients. But each meal also includes a few bitter astringent, pungent, light, dry, and cold ingredients, no matter what your specific body requires. To achieve balance just eat a bite or two of those tastes or qualities that increase Vata, but make the foods that are best for your own balance the main part of the meal. Eating in a balanced way brings feelings of satisfaction.

## Cooking and Eating Tips for Vata

- Heat food thoroughly, serve promptly.
- Eat warm, well-cooked food.
- Drink tepid or warm liquids during and at the end of the    meal, layering solid food with liquid.
- Always eat bread spread with ghee,butter, or nut butters—never dry.
- Cook all vegetables until soft.
- Serve all soups—including lentil and bean soups—in a very liquid consistency.
- Prepare cooked cereals and grains with milk rather than water.
- Serve tossed green salads without raw vegetables.
- Do not serve dried out  or leftover cooked food.
- Serve soft, ripe fruit
- Do not eat while standing up, driving, talking on the phone, or watching television.

### In Vata's Pantry

Here are some commonly used, less perishable foods for Vata-balanced cooking. These items can be kept on hand year round and used as needed everyday.

| | |
|---|---|
| Spices: | asafoetida (hing), caraway, cardamom, cinnamon, cloves, cumin, ginger, licorice root powder, mustard seed, Vata churna, pepper, salt. |
| Herbs: | basil, dill, fennel, parsley, saffron, savory, tarragon. |
| Grains & Others: | rice, wheat flours, lentils, ghee and cooking oils, sugar, honey, molasses, dates, raisins, figs, coconut, sweet potatoes, nuts and nut butters. |

## About the Recipes

Although the recipes and sample menu in this chapter are especially good for maintaining Vata in balance, many of these recipes can be prepared for a meal to serve to people with different dietary needs. Many times a recipe that is good for one body type is also good for others. When using AyurVedic menu planning principles it is difficult to create recipes exclusively for one constituion because so much in life is good for everyone. At a meal offering a variety of dishes, each person would simply select the amount from each that is best for him. Because some of these recipes are useful for more than the Vata constitution, they may appear—sometimes with minor changes—in Pitta or Kapha sections of this book as well. All the recipes that appear anywhere in this book are collected in Chapter 10, "An Ayurveda Recipe Companion."

## Main Points in AyurVedic Menu Planning

- Present all tastes and qualities.

- Order of the meal: begin on time with an appetizer.

- Alternate heavy and light foods throughout the meal.

- Use color, texture, and delicious flavors to stimulate the eye and palate.

## About the Vata Menu

A well-balanced Vata menu will have a great number of salty, sour, sweet tastes and  more rich, heavy , oily (unctuous), hot qualities. Vata menus start with a good appetizer and end with a mouthwatering dessert.

The following sample menu makes a rather elaborate meal if everything on the menu were prepared. If the heavy sweet desserts seem too filling, a simple fruit salad could conclude the meal. This menu is an example of a Vata-reducing meal, not an absolute plan to follow. The predominant tastes and qualities of each selection are noted.

The relish tray is of particular interest in this meal. It presents  a variety of sweet, sour , salty, and pungent  little appetizers that invite Vata to nibble just enough to spark digestion, but not dull the appetite.

## A Sample Vata Menu

RELISH TRAY
PICKLES * OLIVES * CHEESES * DIPS * SAUCES * SPREADS
(Sweet , Sour, Pungent, Salty)

GINGER CARROT SOUP
(Pungent, Sweet, Oily, Salty, Hot)

ASPARAGUS SALAD
with RASPBERRY VINAIGRETTE
(Sweet, Bitter, Slightly Sour and Astringent, Cold)

RICH STUFFED GREEN PEPPERS
(Sweet, Salty, Heavy, Oily)
or
ZUCCHINI AND TOMATO FRY
(Sweet, Sour, Bitter, Slightly Pungent, Oily)

SQUASH ROLLS WITH BUTTER
(Sweet, Slightly Salty, Oily)

CREAMY RICE PUDDING
(Sweet, Heavy)
and/or
CHOCOLATE CUSTARD PIE
(Sweet, Heavy)

## Curried Herb Cheese Dip

A sour, pungent little dip to serve with crackers, chips, or raw vegetables.

Makes 1 cup

    1/2 cup sour cream
    1/2 cup ricotta cheese
    1 tablespoon lemon juice
    3 tablespoons parsley, minced
    1 tablespoon basil, minced
    1/2 teaspoon dry mustard
    1/2 teaspoon paprika
    1/4 teaspoon ground white pepper
    A pinch cayenne pepper
    1/2 teaspoon cumin seeds

In a small bowl cream sour cream and cheese thoroughly. Mix in lemon juice, parsley, basil, mustard, paprika, and peppers. Roast cumin seeds in a hot iron pan until just turning color, then grind finely and add to mixture.

Spoon into serving bowl, cover, and chill in refrigerator for two or three hours to set the flavors.

## Pineapple Ginger-Cream Spread

This sweet, pungent, and sour little sandwich spread is best for Vata but both Pitta and Kapha can enjoy some spread on a cracker or two. This makes a fine celery stuffing for a party relish tray.

Makes 1 cup

    8 ounces cream cheese
    1/4 cup fresh ginger, chopped
    2 1/2 tablespoons crushed pineapple, drained
    1/2 teaspoon nutmeg
    1/4 teaspoon cardamom, ground

Mix all ingredients together thoroughly. Cover and set aside in refrigerator an hour before serving.

## Ginger Carrot Soup

A pungent, sweet, oily, and salty soup that is a good appetizer for Vata, this is a great soup to serve as part of a light meal on a "winter-almost-spring" day. It begins with a basic Vata broth that serves as a basis for many other Vata-balancing main dish recipes, gravies, and sauces.

Serves 6 to 8

    2 cups Vata Broth (recipe follows)
    2 cups milk
    2 tablespoons ghee
    2 teaspoons sugar
    1/4 teaspoon pepper
    1/2 teaspoon cardamom
    1/4 cup chopped fresh ginger
    2 cups shredded carrots
    Juice of 1/2 orange
    1/2 to 3/4 cup  heavy cream
    Butter as garnish

Bring broth and milk to a boil in a heavy  2-quart pan.  Add ghee, sugar, pepper, and cardamom. Stir and cook for a minute over moderately high heat. Add ginger and cook for an additional 2 or 3 minutes until you can  smell the ginger clearly. Stir in carrots and orange juice. Simmer over low heat, stirring frequently for about an hour until carrots are pulpy.

Turn off heat. Cover and let the flavors blend while cooling. When ready to serve purée in a food mill or food processor for about 1minute. Then return to the pot. Reheat just to boiling point and reduce to simmer. Add cream. If it seems too thick add a little water. To further enrich the soup, a pat of butter can be floated  on top of each bowl while serving.

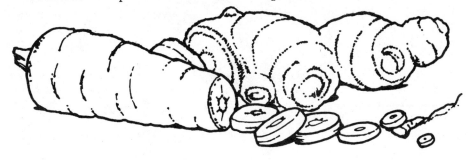

## Vata Broth

2 quarts boiling water
1 teaspoon salt
1/2 teaspoon pepper
Choose at least three different Vata-reducing vegetables, herbs, and spices from this list:

1 cup carrots, sliced
1/2 cup tomatoes, chopped
1/2 cup parsley, chopped
1/2 cup celery, diced
1 cup green beans, cut in inch pieces
1 bay leaf
1/2 teaspoon crushed fenugreek
1/4 teaspoon crumbled saffron
1/2 teaspoon ground cumin
2 tablespoons Vata Churna can be added, or to taste
1 tablespoon ghee

Bring water to a boil in heavy pan. Add the salt, pepper, and vegtables. Simmer covered for 15 minutes. Then add the remaining ingredients. Stir, undisturbed half an hour. Strain vegetables and use the broth. The vegetables can be eaten separately with a little salt, pepper, and butter.cover, and simmer another 5 minutes. Then turn off the heat and allow to sit

## Asparagus Salad in Raspberry Vinaigrette

A colorful and unusual salad, it is sweet, a little sour, astringent, and heavy.

Serves 4

>  10-12 asparagus stalks
>  4 large lettuce leaves
>  Raspberry vinaigrette
>  Coarsely ground pepper
>  1/2 teaspoon salt

Clean asparagus and steam whole stalks. When tender, yet still a bright green, remove from steamer and immediately blanch in cold water to retain the color. Refrigerate until just cool. When ready to serve, arrange the spears on lettuce leaves. Pour raspberry vinaigrette dressing over the middle of the spears. Sprinkle with salt and coarsely ground pepper.

## Raspberry Vinaigrette

>  2 tablespoons white vinegar
>  1/2 cup light oil, safflower or sunflower
>  1/4 teaspoon salt
>  1 cup of fresh raspberries, washed, or a 10-ounce package of frozen raspberries, defrosted

Mix vinegar, salt, and oil in a jar with tight-fitting lid. Put raspberries in a sieve—or drain frozen raspberries—and purée by mashing against the sides with a wooden spoon. Mix raspberry purée with an equal part of the vinaigrette dressing. Mix very well just before serving.

## Rich Stuffed Peppers

A delicious main dish that is nourishing for Vata with its sweet, salty, bitter, and slightly astringent tastes. This warm, rich, heavy stuffing can be baked separately in a buttered casserole and served as a side dish.

Serves 6

> 3 large green peppers, halved and blanched
> 1/2 cup ghee or butter
> 3/4 cup celery stalks and leaves, chopped
> 2 small zucchini, cubed
> 1/4 cup parsley, chopped
> 1/2 cup sweet red pepper, chopped
> 1/4 cup pecans or cashews, coarsely chopped
> 4 cups soft bread cubes
> 1/2 teaspoon salt
> 1 teaspoon crushed sage
> 1/2 teaspoon thyme
> 1/4 to 1/2 teaspoon coarsely ground pepper

To Blanch Peppers:

Bring 2 quarts of water to a boil. Meanwhile halve peppers and remove seeds and membrane. Drop them into boiling water and allow to boil for 3 minutes. Remove from pot and immediately run under cold water. Drain with hollow side down on a towel until ready to stuff.

For the Stuffing:

Preheat oven to 350°. Heat ghee in a large frying pan or deep pot. Add vegetables and saute, stirring frequently for about 20 minutes or until soft. Add nuts, then breadcubes and seasonings. Toss well and heat through. Mound stuffing into pepper halves and place in lightly oiled 9 x 12 inch baking pan. Bake uncovered for 10 minutes.

## Zucchini and Tomato Fry

A satisfying and colorful main dish with sweet, sour, bitter, salty, and slightly pungent tastes. The oily and heavy qualities are especially good for Vata's nutrition.

Serves 4

> 2 tablespoons ghee
> 1 teaspoon black mustard
> 1 teaspoon cumin seeds, roasted and crushed
> 1 teaspoon coriander, ground
> 1/4 teaspoon fenugreek, ground
> 1 teaspoon turmeric
> 1/2 teaspoon ground ginger
> 4 medium zucchini, peeled, quartered, and sliced thin
> 2 to 3 tomatoes, peeled and sliced
> 1/2 teaspoon salt (or to taste)

Heat ghee in a large frying pan or wok over moderate heat. Add mustard seeds. When they begin to pop add the remaining spices. Stir-fry over low heat for 1 minute. Then add zucchini and increase heat to moderately high. Fry uncovered until just tender. Stir frequently. Add tomatoes and salt. Stir and cook for 3 or 4 minutes more. Serve with rice or pasta.

## A Cooking Tip for Vata

Peel zucchini before using to remove the bitter taste — it will have the same beneficial effect as any other squash.

33

## Squash Rolls

If you have some leftover Ginger Carrot Soup or other thick vegetable soup substitute it for the cooked squash. These rolls are sweet, oily, a little heavy, and they are very moist and tender.

Makes 1 1/2 dozen

> 1/3 cup ghee or butter
> 1 cup milk
> 1/2 teaspoon crushed saffron
> 1/4 teaspoon nutmeg
> 1/4 teaspoon ground cardamom
> 1/3 cup brown or white sugar
> 1 cup yellow squash, cooked and pureed
> 1 package dry yeast
> 1/4 cup warm water
> 6 to 7 cups unbleached flour

Preheat oven to 375°.

In a saucepan heat ghee, milk, saffron, spices, and sugar. Bring to boiling point. Remove from heat, stir in squash purée. Let cool.

In a large bowl dissolve yeast in very warm water (100°) and wait 2 to 3 minutes for it to foam. Pour in the warm (not hot) squash mixture. Then begin stirring the flour into the squash, a cup at a time, until the dough starts to come away from the sides of the bowl. It will be very soft and tender to the touch.

Turn dough out on floured board, rub your hands with ghee or oil, and knead about 5 minutes until the dough is smooth and not too sticky to handle. Add flour as needed. Let it rest while you wash and oil the bowl. Put the dough in the bowl and turn it to coat with oil. Cover with plastic wrap or a damp towel and let rise in a warm place for 45 minutes to an hour or until doubled. Push dough down gently and turn out on floured board. Shape golf-ball-size pieces into rolls. Do not stretch them too much to avoid tearing. Place on greased baking sheet. If sides are touching, softer rolls result. Rolls placed one inch apart on the sheet makes them crispier. Cover with a damp towel and let rise until doubled (about 40 minutes) or they are the size you want. Bake 15 to 20 minutes until just golden brown on top. Remove and brush with ghee. Serve warm.

## Creamy Rice Pudding

This rich, nourishing dessert is sweet, heavy, and slightly pungent. Rice pudding and other milk-based puddings are best for digestion when served warm. Long, slow cooking over low heat allows the rice grains to blend so well with the other ingredients that it becomes a creamy, easily digested treat.

Serves 4 to 6

> 3 cups water
> 2 cinnamon sticks
> 1 cup long grain rice
> 3 cups warm milk
> 1 cup sugar
> 1/2 cup raisins
> 1/4 teaspoon crumbled saffron threads
> 1/2 cup blanched almonds, finely chopped

Bring the water and cinnamon sticks to a boil in a large pot. Add the rice and simmer on low, covered, for about 15 to 20 minutes or until the water evaporates and the rice is soft. Meanwhile, mix the milk, sugar, raisins, saffron, and almonds in a bowl and set aside.

When the rice is soft, add the milk mixture to the pot and cook over moderately high heat until just boiling. Reduce heat to low and allow to simmer, uncovered, 20 to 30 minutes. Stir frequently. The pudding is done when everything is well blended and the rice grains can barely be seen. Pour into dishes and serve warm.

## Chocolate Custard Pie

This delicious, sweet, unctuous (oily), astringent, bitter filling decreases Vata. It is also good for increasing weight.

Make one 9-inch pie

9-inch pre-baked pie crust
1 pint half-and-half cream
1 pint whipping cream
1/4 cup cornstarch
1/2 cup sugar
6 oz. semi-sweet chocolate chips
1/2 teaspoon vanilla
1/4 cup choclate chips
1 cup sweetened whipped cream
Shaved bitter chocolate (optional)

In a small bowl mix cornstarch and sugar together and set aside. Heat creams over low heat or in the top of a double boiler. Add small amount of hot cream to the dry ingredients and whisk to blend. When smooth, pour slowly into the rest of the cream, whisking all the time. Stir constantly until thickened. Remove from heat and add 6 ounces chocolate chips and vanilla. Stir until blended. Cover with plastic wrap directly on filling and refrigerate until cold.

Meanwhile bake pie shell. When it comes out of the  oven spread with remaining chocolate chips evenly on the bottom and let cool. If chips do not melt entirely slip the pan back in the turned off oven for a minute or two.

When ready to serve, fill cooled pie shell with the custard and top with whipped cream and chocolate shavings.

## Other Recipes Especially for Vata

When planning other menus try any of these recipes appropriate for a Vata diet. They can be found in Chapter 10, "An AyurVeda Recipe Companion." Some of them may also appear in the Pitta and Kapha chapters or elsewhere in this book with minor variations .

## Beverages

Bed and Breakfast Drink
Fragrantly Spiced Lassi
Plain Lassi
Saffron Milk Tea
Three-in-One Samhita Supreme
Watermelon-Strawberry Punch

## Appetizers

Cheese Crackers
Golden Panir Cubes
Golden Yummies

## Salads

Macedonia di Fruita
Splendid Garden Salad
Tossed Green Salad

## Dressings, Sauces, Dips, Spreads, and Marinades

Avocado Cheese Sauce and Dip
Basic Cheese Sauce
Cream Tahini Sauce
Deanna's Vinaigrette
Ginger Soy Gravy
Herbed Vinaigrette
Pitta Churna Salad Dressing and Marinade
Scrumptious Sesame Orange Dressing and Sauce
Simple Vinaigrette Dressing

## Other Basics

Ghee
Panir and Ricotta Soft Cheese

## Breads

Cornbread
French Bread
Little Flat Breads
Puris And Chapatis
Squash Rolls

## Soups

Baked Lentil Soup
Potage Printanier
Sweet Potato Soup
Vegetable Soup with Fresh Herbs

## Main Dishes

Artichokes Stuffed with Herbed Cheese
Curried Vegtables and Panir
Fagioloni in Umido Volponi
Fried-Spiced Potatoes
Moroccan Delight with Couscous
Oven Baked French Fries
Pasta and Green Sauce
Petis Pois Braise Laitue
Rice Pilaf
Saffron Rice
Stuffed Shells with Artichoke Cream Sauce
Sweet Summer Curry
Tofu Nut Burgers
Vegetables & Brown Rice Sauté
Whole Grain Vegeatable Sauté

## Side Dishes (part of a main meal)

Baked Wild Rice Casserole
Green and Gold Squash
Layered Vegetable Loaf
Simple Baked Carrots

## Desserts

Almond Custard Fresh Fruit Pie
American Apple Pie
Apple Dumplings
Fresh Ginger Cookies
Fruit Shortcake
Italian Hazelnut Cookies
Jam Diagonals
Kaffa's Dream
Lemon Scones
Lemony Date Bars
Marble Cake with Vanilla Sauce and English Cream
Oatmeal Raisin Cookies
Old Fashioned Tea Cake
R&S Couscous
Rich Chocolate Mousse
Strawberry Yogurt Pie Filling
Super Chocolate Brownies
Swedish Chocolate Cream Pie
Sweet Chocolate Cake With Cherry Sauce
Sweet Fruit and Spice Bread
Sweet Potato Apple Pie
White Figs in Apricot Sauce

## For a Vata-Balancing Diet

**FAVOR**

General: Increased quantity of food, Oily (Unctuous), Warm Food and Drinks, Heavy, Heating Food, Sweet, Sour, and Salty Tastes

Dairy: All Dairy Products

Sweeteners: Any Sugar, Honey, Molasses

Oils: All Oils, especially Ghee

Grains: Rice, Wheat, Rye, Oats

Beans: Mung and Urad Lentils, Tofu

Fruits: Grapes, Cherries, Peaches, Melons, Avocado, Coconut, Banana, Orange, Pineapple, Plums, Berries, Mango, Papaya, Olives, Lemon, Lime

Vegetables: Beets, Carrots, Asparagus, Cucumber, Sweet Potato, Avocado, Artichoke, Tomato, Peppers

Spices: Asafoetida (Hing), Basil, Black Pepper, Caraway, Cardamom, Cinnamon, Clove, Cumin, Garlic, Ginger, Mustard, Poppyseed, Salt

Nuts: Any Except Walnuts

Beverages: Tepid Water, Fruit and Vegetable juice, Warm Milk, Herbal Teas

Animal Food For Non-Vegetarians: Chicken, Turkey, Seafood


**REDUCE**

General: Light Diet, Dry Foods, Cold Food and Drinks
Pungent, Bitter, and Astringent Tastes

Grains: Large Amounts of Barley, Corn, Millet, Buckwheat

Fruits: Apple, Cranberries, Unripe fruit

Vegetables: Peas, Green Leafy Vegetables, Broccoli, Cabbage, Cauliflower, Zucchini, Potato, or Raw Vegetables, Most Sprouted Legumes/Seeds/Beans

Spices: Allspice, Coriander, Nutmeg, Turmeric, Oregano

Nuts: Walnuts

Beans: All Beans Except Soy (Tofu) and Lentils

Beverages: Iced Drinks, Carbonated Drinks, Thick Milkshakes, Coffee, Black Tea

Animal Food For Non-Vegetarians: Beef

# Chapter 3

# Cooking for Pitta

## What is Pitta?

Of the three basic constitutions Pitta is most like fire. It is hot, dry, and light. Your nature is most like Pitta if many of the characteristics in this list best describe you:

## Pitta Characteristics

| Balanced | Out of Balance |
|---|---|
| Enterprising, idealist | Pressures self and others |
| Energetic, organized | Too time-conscious, excited |
| Often charismatic leader | Task-oriented, critical |
| Lively, friendly | Irritable, quick tempered |
| Curious, broad interests | Activity overload |
| Radiant, warm skin, freckles | Blemishes, gray hair |
| Good appetite and digestion | Ulcers, stomach upsets |

## The Best Diet For Pitta

For most of the year but especially in hot weather, Pitta should follow a cooling, sweet, and nourishing diet. Pitta-increasing foods are best enjoyed in the winter, and then only in moderation. Those with Pitta-Kapha or Kapha-Pitta constitutions follow the Pitta-balancing diet in summer and Kapha-balancing diet during cold weather, as described in Chapter 4, "Cooking for Kapha." Those with Vata-Pitta and Pitta-Vata imbalances usually follow a Pitta-decreasing diet in summer and Vata-balancing diet the rest of the time.

## General Pitta Diet

### Favor

- Cool Food and Drinks
- Tastes: Sweet, Bitter, Astringent
- Qualities: Heavy, Cold, Oily
- Moderate Amounts of Substantial Meals
- Salads
- Rich Food

### Reduce

- Hot Foods and Drinks
- Tastes: Pungent, Sour, Salty
- Qualities: Light, Hot, Dry
- Light and Infrequent Meals

## Tastes and Qualities Best for Pitta

A properly balanced meal for Pitta types contains foods with all of the six tastes and six food qualities, but those following a Pitta-balancing diet should make most of their meal from those ingredients that reduce Pitta.

# Best Food Tastes for Pitta

• Sweet  • Bitter  • Astringent •

## Menu Planning For Pitta

People with outstanding Pitta characteristics are naturally warm, even in winter. They are most like a hot summer day, so menus for Pitta types during summer and into early autumn include a greater proportion of moist and cooling foods and less protein. A Pitta-balancing diet is abundant in seasonal fruits and vegetables. Almost all of the fruits and vegetables available during the hot months pacify Pitta.

# Best Food Qualities for Pitta

## • Heavy • Oily • Cold •

Care should be taken not to exclusively eat fruits and light foods in the summer. Foods with heavier, oily qualities than are found in most fruits need to be included in all main meals. Typically, Pitta has a strong appetite requiring satisfying meals that include such wheat products as pasta, breads, and rolls. Other ingredients with heavy qualities—rice, artichokes, potatoes, and tofu are a few standards.Especially good news for those on a Pitta-balancing diet is that they do not need to skip sweet desserts. Since sugar and other naturally sweet foods pacify Pitta, desserts are an important part of each main meal.

## Main Points in AyurVedic Menu Planning

- Present all tastes and qualities

- Order of the meal: begin on time with appetizer

- Alternate heavy and light foods throughout the meal

- Use color, texture, and delicious flavors to stimulate the eye and palate

## Seasonal Menu Changes

Drinking lots of water and cooling drinks, particularly sweet fruit juices, is most refreshing for Pitta in the summer. For those following a Pitta-reducing diet in the winter and early spring, fresh sweet fruits and cooling vegetables are still important, but also more of the warm soups and higher protein entrees we associate with cold winter days can appear on the menu.

*There is no need for watermelon in the winter.*
*Your body needs watery food in the summer.*
*Nature grows foods according to the correct*
*season for you.*
*We must think more about Nature when we*
*plan our meals.*

-Dr. P. D. Subhedar

## Maintaining Pitta's Good Digestion

Those with a Pitta constitution rarely need appetizers to stimulate agni. Their digestive fires are usually ready when the food is. But maintaining the good digestion of those following a Pitta-balancing diet depends on eating at regular times, eating when hungry, and, as far as possible, not postponing meals. Pitta types not only become irritable when overly hungry, but they tend to eat too much too quickly without enjoying the meal. This results in feelings of dissatisfaction or discomfort after eating.

## Cooking/Eating Tips For Pitta

• Pitta most appreciates cool, rather substantial or heavy, rich-tasting soups, appetizers, and main dishes served in moderate portions.

• Light foods such as tossed salads or dishes of millet and barley should make up less than one third of a meal.

• Serve mostly warm to cool foods rather than steaming hot ones.

• Use varieties of sweet fruits in mixed casseroles with vegetables, rice, and in other grains.

• When following new recipes reduce salt by one half.

• Substitute 2 tablespoons yogurt for each egg in baking recipes, and increase leavening slightly.

• Sip tepid or slightly chilled drinks with a meal, rather than iced ones.

• Serve a salad of leafy greens daily.

• Rarely cook with tomatoes, cheese, yogurt, sour cream, or pungent spices.

• Instead of pungent or frankly fiery spices use ground licorice root, cinnamon, coriander, nutmeg, and fresh cooling herbs.

• Do not serve leftovers from the day before.

• Do not prepare food or eat when upset, angry, or agitated.

• Sit down to eat in a settled, undisturbed atmosphere.

• End a meal with a sweet dessert or fresh sweet fruit.

## In Pitta's Pantry

Here are some less perishable foods frequently used when cooking for Pitta types or in the hot weather of Pitta season. These staples can be kept in stock all the time and replenished as needed.

| | |
|---|---|
| Spices: | anise seeds, cardamom, cinnamon, coriander, licorice root, mace, nutmeg, poppy seeds, paprika, turmeric, Pitta churna |
| Herbs: | dill, fennel, parsley, savory, tarragon |
| Grains & Others: | ghee, rice, wheat flour, sugar, dried fruit, walnuts, cashews, unblanched almonds, nut butters, lentils, sunflower or safflower oil |

## About the Sample Menu

The sample menu in this chapter is especially good for those who want to balance Pitta dosha. It is a good example of an AyurVedic menu because all six tastes and food qualities are included. But the larger amounts of sweet, astringent, bitter tastes and the heavy, oily, and cold qualites best suit Pitta diets. Because many of the recipes are good for balancing other body types as well, they may be appear in recipe lists for Vata or Kapha. All the recipes for all constitutional types used in this book are collected in Chapter 10 "An AyurVeda Recipe Companion."

## A Sample Pitta Menu

POMEGRANATE JUICE with MINT LEAF GARNISH
(Sweet, Astringent, Sour, Slightly Pungent, Cold)

SUMMER GARDEN SOUP
(Sweet, Bitter, Astringent, Heavy, Cold)

MOROCCAN DELIGHT
(All Tastes, Heavy, Oily)

SPLENDID LAYERS SALAD
(Sweet, Bitter, Astringent, Oily, Heavy)
Or
COLESLAW WITH CARAWAY DRESSING

(Sweet, Sour, Salty, Bitter, Dry, Astringent),

LITTLE FLAT BREADS
(Sweet, Slightly Bitter and Salty, Heavy)

PINEAPPLE ICE
(Sweet, Cold)

OATMEAL RAISIN COOKIES
(Sweet, Slightly Salty, Heavy)

## Creamy Summer Garden Soup

A sweet, slightly bitter, and astringent soup this is both refreshing in summer and good for reducing Pitta. Use water or Pitta broth as the basic soup stock. This broth can serve as a start to many Pitta-reducing sauces, gravies, and marinades.

Serves 6 to 8

2 cups Swiss chard, chopped
2 small zucchini, thinly sliced
1 cup Bok Choy or Swiss chard leaves, chopped
2 quarts Pitta Broth—see next recipe
1 teaspoon French tarragon, minced
1 tablespoon ghee
1 very ripe avocado, mashed
1 cup heavy cream
1/2 cup shredded raw beets or shredded red cabbage
8 to 10 sprigs fresh fennel or dill

Steam vegetables for 12 minutes or until zucchini is very soft; or cook in pressure cooker for 4 minutes. Cool slightly and puree in food processor or blender until creamy.

Heat Pitta broth in large heavy pot and add vegtable puree. Simmer and stir until well blended. In a separate saucepan heat cream. When just beginning to boil reduce heat and add tarragon, ghee, and mashed avocado. Stir very well and fold into vegetable soup. Cool for an hour, then chill for at least three hours before serving.

Serve in a large decorative glass bowl with shredded beet or cabbage garnish and herbs. Or garnish each bowl individually as you serve.

Note: Recipe can be cut in half if you are cooking for less than 6 persons with Pitta dosha.

## Basic Pitta Broth

Pitta broth, a combination of Pitta-reducing vegetables, herbs, and spices, is a basic soup stock. The flavor of the broth will vary depending on the combination of ingredients selected. When making this broth choose at least three different Pitta-reducing vegetables, herbs, and spices. Pitta broth is useful as a gravy base or for the beginning of a vegetable cream sauce. It is also a refreshing drink for Pitta when served chilled with a celery stick and a garnish of fresh fennel or dill.

Makes about 2 quarts

2 quarts water
1 cup broccoli, chopped
1 cup green beans, chopped
1 cup potatoes, peeled and diced
1/2 teaspoon salt
1/4 teaspoon pepper, white or black
2 tablespoons Pitta Churna
            or
2 teaspoons ground coriander
1/2 teaspoon crushed anise seed
3 or 4 crushed green cardamom pods
1 tablespoon ghee (optional)

In a large pot of boiling salted water add vegetables. Turn to low, cover and simmer for 15 minutes. Stir in remaining ingredients. Adding a tablespoon of ghee makes a richer broth. Cover and simmer 5 more minutes. Then turn off heat and let pot sit undisturbed for 30 minutes. Strain and use the broth. The cooked vegetables can be pureed and used in a creamy soup, or they can be simply eaten with a little butter.

## Moroccan Delight

An elaborate and beautiful dish to serve at a party. This recipe combines ingredients that reduce Pitta. The "delight" comes from savoring a large variety of stimulating flavors and exotic color. By preparing groups of ingredients separately, the tastes remain distinct from one another even after they are finally combined before serving. A little of every taste is represented, but it is mostly sweet in taste and heavy and oily in qualitiy.

Serves 4 to 6 generously

2 cups marinated tofu
2 cups broccoli flowerets
2 cups cauliflowerets
1 large sweet pimento pepper, cut in bite-size pieces
1 can (8-ounces) artichoke hearts, not marinated, quartered
Ghee
2 tablespoons olive oil, or other cooking oil
1/2 cup warm water
1/2 teaspoon ground coriander
1 tablespoon turmeric
1 teaspoon ground cardamom
1/2 teaspoon to 1 teaspoon salt, to taste
1/2 cup bright orange dried apricots, sliced
1/4 cup pitted dates, chopped
6 cups cooked couscous or rice
1/4 cup blanched almonds, sliced

To Marinate Tofu:

Marinate tofu at least 2 hours before you are ready to cook.

1 quart sweet red fruit juice, such as raspberry, pomegranate, plum, strawberry or a blend of these
1/4 teaspoon each nutmeg, ground coriander, and cinnamon
1 tablespoon tamari
1 pound firm tofu—with water pressed out and cubed

## Moroccan Delight, continued

In a 2-quart saucepan heat the juice, spices, and tamari. Remove from heat and mix in the tofu cubes. Cover and marinate for 2 or 3 hours at room temperature, or overnight in the refrigerator. For a quick marinade omit the spices and simply pour juice and tamari mixture over the tofu. Cover and set aside for at least 2 hours.

When ready to prepare drain the tofu. Steam broccoli and cauliflower for 10 minutes. Set aside.

To Prepare:

Heat 3 tablespoons ghee in a wok or heavy frying pan and saute tofu cubes until they are lightly browned—about 10 minutes. Set aside in a large bowl. In the same pan heat 1 tablespoon of ghee over medium heat. Add sesame seeds and stir until they begin to turn brown and start popping.

Immediately add red pepper pieces and artichoke hearts. Sauté for 2 minute, tossing to cover the vegetables with the seeds. Then gently mix in with the tofu. Set aside and cover. Again in the same pan heat 2 tablespoons of oil over medium heat. Then add turmeric, coriander, cardamom, and salt. Stir until turmeric lumps disappear. Then slowly stir in 1/2 cup warm water. This makes a golden sauce.

Add steamed broccoli and cauliflower. Stir until cauliflower is uniformly golden, then add apricots and dates. Add more water as needed to keep the sauce from drying out. Simmer over low heat for another minute, stirring frequently. Then gently fold in the tofu cubes and stir-fry another minute or 2 until they are dark brown. Arrange on a bed of steaming couscous or rice and sprinkle with almonds.

If not serving immediately, cover tightly and keep warm in 200° oven.

To prepare this dish for a celebration or large party, allow 1/2 cup tofu and 1/2 cup vegetables per person. For an authentic ethnic touch, serve with Little Flat Breads or pita bread.

## Splendid Layers Salad

A layered, rather "thick" salad that is good at a picnic or served as a light meal on a summer evening. The tastes are sweet, bitter, astringent, and slightly salty. It has oily, cold, and heavy qualities. This combination is good for Pitta types since the heavier vegetables provide enough substance for Pitta's healthy appetite. When eaten in small amounts this salad is all right for Vata, but the cold and heavy qualities aggravate Kapha Be sure to cut everything into bite-size pieces when preparing. Each vegetable can be cut in a different shape to add visual interest.

Serves 6 to 8

2 heads of bibb lettuce
1/2 head red cabbage, shredded
6 large artichoke hearts, steamed and quartered
          or
Prepared artichokes: 14-ounce can, drained and quartered or
     10 ounces frozen, defrosted and quartered
1 pound asparagus, cut in 1-inch pieces and steamed
1 cucumber, washed, scored with tines of fork, sliced very thin
1 medium jicama or 3 sunchokes, cut in triangular shapes and sliced
4 tablespoons Pitta Churna Salad Dressing (recipe follows)
4 large leaves Romaine lettuce, de-ribbed, cut in 1 inch squares
1 tablespoon fresh mint, dill, and/or fennel
1/3 cup curly parsley leaves, broken in clusters
1/4 cup small seedless grapes or raisins
1 cup mixed salad greens, as available, such as arugula, beet leaves, hon
     tsai tai, chicory, escarole torn or chopped in small pieces
1 red apple, cored and diced
1/4 cup croutons, toasted

To Assemble:

Line the bottom and sides of a deep, straight-sided glass bowl or saladbowl with Bibb lettuce leaves. Sprinkle with enough red cabbage to cover the bottom. Layer with about one third of the "thick" ingredients: artichoke hearts, asparagus, cucumber, and jicama. Pour one tablespoon Pitta Churna Dressing over this layer. Begin next layer with a sprinkling of red cabbage and Romaine pieces about an inch thick.

## Splendid Layers Salad, continued

Spread on half of the chopped fresh herbs. Arrange another third of the "thick" ingredients and add the grapes or raisins. Sprinkle with a little red cabbage for color and pour on one tablespoon Pitta Churna dressing to end this layer. Then cover the surface with mixed chopped greens. Sprinkle with the remaining cabbage, herbs, the last third of the vegetables, diced apple, and remaining salad dressing in that order. Ring the outside with parsley clusters and sprinkle croutons in the center. Be sure the bibb lettuce lines the edges of the bowl attractively. Add more leaves, if necessary, to fill in empty spaces. Cover and refrigerate one or two hours before serving.

## Pitta Churna Dressing

Pitta Churna, an AyurVedic blend of herbs and spices especially good for those following a Pitta diet, is useful in soups, dressings, and vegetable and fruit dishes.

    1/2 cup oil, sunflower or safflower
    2 tablespoons warm water
    1 1/2 to 2 teaspoons Pitta Churna
    1/2 teaspoon salt
    2 tablespoons vinegar

Place all ingredients in a jar or blender. Cover tightly and blend well. Let mixture stand for 5 to 10 minutes and blend again. Shake well before serving.

## Coleslaw with Caraway Dressing

A basic "cold" salad for Pitta, it can even be eaten in winter when cabbage is at its best. This salad adds the sour taste to Pitta's diet and should be served as part of a balanced meal that includes other Pitta-reducing dishes, rather than being eaten by itself.

Makes 4 to 6 servings

    1 teaspoon caraway seeds
    1/4 cup sour cream
    1/8 cup plain yogurt
    1 teaspoon sugar
    1/2 teaspoon vinegar
    1/2 medium head cabbage, finely shredded

In a small heavy pan toast the caraway seeds over a low flame. Stir constantly until lightly brown. Remove from heat and crush with mortar and pestle or in a spice grinder. Whisk sour cream, yogurt, and sugar in a small bowl. Add the caraway and vinegar. Then toss thoroughly with the shredded cabbage. Cover and chill for at least an hour before serving.

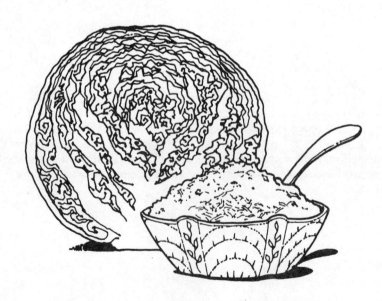

## Little Flat Breads

These chewy disks are good as "food pushers" to accompany Moroccan Delight or other vegetable dishes, or even as a breakfast bread. They are sweet and slightly bitter.

Makes 8 small disks

1 package dry yeast
1 1/2 cups warm water
2 tablespoons oil or ghee
1 teaspoon salt
1 cup whole wheat flour
3 to 4 cups white flour
4 tablespoons poppy seeds

In a large bowl dissolve yeast in warm water. When it is frothy stir in oil, salt, and whole wheat flour. Begin adding white flour, a cup at a time until a stiff dough is formed. Turn out on a floured surface and wash the bowl.

Oil your hands a little and knead the dough for about 10 minutes, adding small amounts of flour as necessary to make it smooth and elastic. Return the kneaded dough to the bowl. Cover with plastic wrap or a damp towel and place in a warm spot to rise. In about an hour to 1 1/2 hours it will be doubled in bulk.

Oil 2 baking sheets. Preheat oven to 450°.

If using sesame seeds, roast them in a heavy skillet over low heat until they are just light brown and starting to pop. Set aside.

Turn dough out on clean work surface. Oil your hands. Punch it down and divide into 8 equal parts. Press each part into a circle with a thin middle and higher outer lip. They will look like little pie crusts. Mark the centers a few times with the tines of a fork. Brush with water and sprinkle some seeds on each disk, pressing the seeds lightly into the dough. Place them on 2 oiled baking sheets, not touching each other.

Bake 10 minutes or until just brown. They are best when eaten warm.

## Pineapple Ice

A perfect dessert for Pitta, especially on a hot day. Sweet, ripe pineapple is especially calming to Pitta. Easy to make and so like authentic Italian ices, a bowl of Pineapple Ice makes a fine ending to an Italian meal.

Makes 1 1/2 quarts

1/4 -1/2 cup sugar, to taste
2 cups water
2 cups fresh pineapple, cored and chopped,
   or
a 14 ounce can of crushed pineapple
1/4 cup lemon juice

Boil the water and sugar in a heavy saucepan for 4 to 5 minutes, stirring until sugar is dissolved. Remove from heat, stir in pineapple and lemon juice. Cool and pour in a shallow bowl. Put in freezer. Every half hour remove and stir vigorously. When about half frozen, whip with an electric mixer, on medium, for one minute. Freeze until firm.

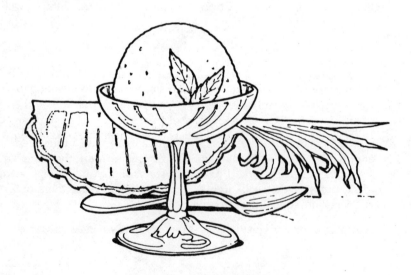

## Oatmeal Raisin Cookies

Highly nutritious and tasty, these cookies ship well and are very good for dunking. Both Vata and Pitta can eat these sweet, heavy, slightly salty cookies.

Makes 4 to 5 dozen

1/3 cup oil
1/2 cup margarine or butter
1 cup white sugar
1 cup brown sugar, packed
1/3 cup milk
2 teaspoons vanilla
1 1/2 cups white flour
1 cup whole wheat flour
1 teaspoon baking powder
1 teaspoon baking soda
1 teaspoon salt
3 cups oats
1 cup raisins
1/2 cup walnuts, broken

Preheat oven to 350°.

Cream margarine and oil. Then add sugars and cream well. Add milk and vanilla. In a separate bowl mix together flour, baking soda, baking powder, and salt. Stir into sugar mixture. Add oats, raisins, and nuts. Mix with fingers if it's too thick to stir. Shape into balls and flatten slightly. Place close together, but not touching, on greased baking sheets. Bake 15 minutes until cookies just turn brown underneath.

# 3 The AyurVeda Cookbook

## Other Recipes Especially Good for Pitta

When planning other menus try any of these recipes appropriate for a Pitta-balancing diet. They can be found in Chapter 10, "An AyurVeda Recipe Companion." Some of them may also appear in the Vata and Kapha chapters or elsewhere in this book with minor variations.

## Beverages

Bed and Breakfast Drink
Fragrantly Spiced Lassi
Pineapple Mint Tea
Plain Lassi
Rose-Petal Milkshake
Sweet Fruit Smoothies
Three-in-One Samhita Supreme
Watermelon-Strawberry Punch

## Appetizers

Cheese Crackers
Golden Panir Cubes
Golden Yummies

## Salads

Asparagus in Raspberry Vinaigrette
Macedonia di Fruita
Tossed Green Salad

## Dressings, Sauces, Spreads, and Marinades

Avocado Cheese Sauce and Dip
Basic Cheese Sauce
Cream Tahini Sauce
Deanna's Vinaigrette
Ginger Soy Gravy
Herbed Vinaigrette
Pineapple Ginger-Cream Spread
Scrumptious Sesame Orange Dressing and Sauce
Simple Vinaigrette Dressing

## Other Basics
Ghee
Panir and Ricotta Soft Cheese

## Bread
French Bread
Puris And Chapatis
Squash Rolls

## Soups
Baked Lentil Soup
Potage Printanier
Sweet Potato Soup
Vegetable Soup with Fresh Herbs

## Main Dishes
Fagioloni in Umido Volponi
Layered Vegetable Casserole
Quick Vegetable Medley
Vegetables & Whole Grain Sauté
Sweet Summer Curry
Saffron Rice
Tofu Nut Burgers
Oven Baked French Fries
Couscous
Pasta and Green Sauce
Petis Pois Braise Laitue
Rice Pilaf

## Side Dishes ( as part of a main meal)
Fried-Spiced Potatoes
Green and Gold Squash
Spiced and Roasted Barley

## Desserts

Almond Custard Fresh Fruit Pie
American Apple Pie
Apple Pie Filling without Sugar
Apple Dumplings with Vanilla Sauce
Chocolate Custard Pie
Creamy Rice Pudding
Fruit Shortcake
Italian Hazelnut Cookies
Jam Diagonals
Kaffa's Dream
Lemon Scones
Lemony Date Bars
Oatmeal Raisin Cookies
Rich and Quick  Chocolate Mousse
R&S Couscous
Strawberry Yogurt Pie Filling
Super Chocolate Brownies
Sweet Chocolate Cake With Cherry Sauce
Sweet Fruit and Spice Bread
Toasty Cinnamon Bar Cookies
White Figs in Apricot Cream Sauce

# For a Pitta-Balancing Diet

FAVOR:

| | |
|---|---|
| General: | Cool Foods and Drinks, Liquids, Heavy, Oily Foods; Sweet, Bitter, and Astringent Tastes |
| Dairy: | Milk, Butter, Ghee, Cream, Panir (Soft Cheese), Ricotta |
| Sweeteners: | All Sweeteners Except Honey and Molasses |
| Oils: | Sunflower, Coconut, Safflower, Olive |
| Grains: | Wheat, Rice, Oats, Millet |
| Fruits: | Grapes, Cherries, Melons, Avocado, Coconut, Orange (Sweet), Plums (Sweet), Lime, Apple, Peach, Dried Fruit |
| Vegetables: | Asparagus, Cucumber, Cabbage, Potato, Sweet Potato, Green Leafy Vegetables, Broccoli, Cauliflower, Celery, Sprouts, Squash, Green Beans, Beets, Eggplant |
| Beans: | All Beans, Lentils, Tofu |
| Spices: | Anise, Black Pepper—in small quantities, Cardamom, Cinnamon, Coriander, Dill, Fennel, Licorice Root, Nutmeg |
| Nuts: | Blanched Almonds, Walnuts, Cashews |
| Beverages: | Cool Water in large quantities, Sweet Fruit Juices, Mint Teas, Warm or Cool Milk, Milkshakes, Fruit Smoothies |

Animal Foods For Non Vegetarians: Chicken, Turkey

REDUCE:

| | |
|---|---|
| General: | Hot Foods and Drinks,Light, Dry Food; Pungent, Sour, and Salty Tastes |
| Dairy: | Yogurt, Cheese, Sour Cream, Cultured Buttermilk |
| Sweeteners: | Honey and Molasses |
| Oils: | Almond, Sesame, Corn |
| Grains: | Corn, Rye, large amounts Millet, Oats, or Barley |
| Fruits: | Grapefruit, Olives, Papaya, Persimmon, Banana, Orange (Sour), Pineapple (Sour), Plums (Sour), unripe Strawberry |
| Vegetables: | Hot Peppers, Tomato, Carrots, Spinach, |
| Spices: | Allspice, Asafoetida (Hing), Basil, Cayenne, Cloves, Cumin, Fenugreek, Garlic, Ginger, Mustard, Salt, Pepper, Saffron |
| Nuts: | Peanuts, Almonds (Unblanched) |
| Beverages: | Hot Drinks, Lemonade or Sour Drinks, many Herbal Teas, Buttermilk, Lassi, large amounts of Coffee or Black Tea |

Animal Food For Non-Vegetarians: Beef, Seafood, Egg Yolks

## Menu Planning Notes:

# Chapter 4

# Cooking for Kapha

## What is Kapha?

Kapha is most like the earth after a spring rain. As an element it is cold, wet, smooth, and heavy. Your nature is most like Kapha if many of the characteristics in this list best describe you.

# Kapha Characteristics

| Balanced | Out of Balance |
| --- | --- |
| Tranquil, easy going, loving | Depressed, bored |
| Strong , good stamina | Listless, weak |
| Steady, methodical activity | Lethargic, body stiff |
| Large, well-built body | Overweight |
| Plentiful hair, smooth, oily skin | Very oily hair/skin |
| Careful learner, good memory | Disinterested |
| Sleeps soundly and long | Excessive sleeping |
| Slow, regular digestion | Poor appetite |

## The Best Diet for Kapha

One way Kapha types and those on a weight-reducing program can maintain health is by following a Kapha-balancing diet. Visit a qualified AyurVeda physician for other useful suggestions. It may happen that one's constitution is a combination of Kapha with Vata or Kapha with Pitta, or even a mixture of Kapha-Pitta-Vata. In that case follow the other dosha-balancing diet during the proper season, and a Kapha-balancing diet during the cold, wet, rainy weather of spring. Those with all-Kapha natures follow a Kapha-balancing diet all year.

## General Kapha Diet
### Favor

- Warm Food and Drinks
- Tastes-- Pungent, Bitter, Astringent
- Qualities--Light, Dry, Hot
- Light Meals
- Appetizers, Salads, Soups
- Rice Cakes and Crackers

### Reduce

- Cold Food and Drinks
- Rich Desserts
- Heavy Meals, Too Much Food
- Tastes--Sweet, Sour, Salty
- Qualities--Cold, Heavy, Oily
- Snacking Between Meals

## Tastes and Qualities Best for Kapha

Here are the best food tastes and qualities for Kapha body types. All six tastes and six qualities are served in every balanced meal, but Kapha should have most of those that help to maintain Kapha in balance.

# Best Food Tastes for Kapha

• Pungent • Astringent • Bitter •

## Kapha's Diet

Kapha appreciates warm, light, easily and quickly digested foods that are on the dry side People with Kapha chacteristics have strong, well-knit bodies that need fewer body-building foods than either Vata or Pitta types. They most efficiently make use of ingredients that increase weight, muscle, and fat. For the sake of healthy growth and balance, foods with heavier qualities that also build strength should not be completely eliminated from Kapha's diet. Kapha needs to develop and maintain a strong body. Such items as breads, pasta, rice, beans, and rich main dishes and desserts simply need to make up a smaller proportion of any day's menu. Since Kapha types tend to put on fat easily, reducing oily, fatty ingredients, for example, by substituting low-fat milk for whole milk or eating fried foods infrequently, is important for maintaining Kapha's balance.

# Best Food Qualities for Kapha

• Light • Hot • Dry •

## Menu Planning for Kapha

Fortunately, menu planning for Kapha is not entirely a question of "reducing" and "avoiding." Most herbs and spices are beneficial to Kapha. The flavors in main dish casseroles, steamed vegetables, grain dishes, and tossed salads can be enhanced with fresh basil, thyme, tarragon, oregano, and other herbs that Vata and Pitta eat little of.

Cooking for Kapha means having fun experimenting with many subtle flavor combinations popular in the contemporary American light gourmet cuisine. The emphasis is on serving varieties of small to medium portions of elegantly presented preparations filled with many hidden nuances of texture and flaver that delight the palate.

## Balance

The most nutritious meals are interesting and varied.  They do not have to be particularly elaborate, but by using many different seasonings and a wide variety of ingredients that include something of all the six tastes and six qualities, it is easy to serve balanced meals every day. If most of a recipe is made up of weight-reducing or Kapha-decreasing ingredients such as barley, leafy greens, pungent herbs and spices, or lentils, then the addition of sweet red peppers, raisins and dates, or even a tomato—which by themselves increase Kapha— won't change the total Kapha-reducing effect of the dish. And this is a good way to add appetizing colors and some sweet or sour tastes to the meal without having them dominate.

Although a healthy meal emphasizes those tastes and qualities best suited for maintaining Kapha in balance, every meal should include sweet, sour, salty tastes as well as some foods with oily, cold, and heavy qualities.  Kapha can nibble at these.

> *Take food to gain Pure Knowledge.*
> *Gain Pure Knowledge to relieve*
> *All sorrow and unhappiness from life.*
> -The Upanishads

## Balance in the Whole Meal

Although certain foods or recipes increase Kapha when eaten by themselves, their effect is somewhat neutralized when eaten they are eaten moderately as a part of a balanced meal.  The fruit salad "Macedonia di Fruita" from the Italian Menu in Chapter Eight, is an example of balance within the whole meal. Whether served as a salad or dessert, this decorative display of sweet apples and oranges, melons, figs, grapes, dates, and other seasonal fruits is good for all body types.  Individually, each of these fruits increases Kapha.  In fact, the entire salad increases Kapha.  Such a fruit salad is not something that people with Kapha constitutions would eat as a meal by itself or in a large amount; but when served as a part of a balanced meal—that is, with other dishes predominately Kapha-reducing—Macedonia di Fruit is good even for Kapha types.

## Cooking/Eating Tips for Kapha

- Kapha appreciates light, dry, warm foods that are not too sweet, salty, or oily.
- Make some foods that are naturally heavy lighter and easier to digest by heating them. Bring water and milk to a boiling point, then allow to cool before drinking or cooking.
- Lighten rice and other grains by frying them in a small amount of oil until the grains begin to turn a light brown. Then cook as usual.
- When following new recipes try reducing both salt and sugar by one half the amount called for.
- Use corn and barley as grains and baking flours.
- Serve tepid water with meals, but drink nothing for one hour after eating.
- Eat such heavy foods as bananas, milk products, potatoes, and yams with a little honey, black pepper, ginger, or other pungent spices rather than by themselves.
- Avoid between meal snacking to maintain a strong appetite.
- Serve a pungent or sweet appetizer before the main meal.
- Serve small to moderate portions of heavy or filling dishes.
- Eat a tossed salad of mixed leafy greens with a light dressing daily.
- Sit down to eat in a settled atmosphere.

## In Kapha's Pantry

Maintain a year round supply of a selection of non-perishible foods that those with Kapha constitutions and others following weight-reducing diets use daily. To keep the freshest ingredients on hand buy staples in small quantities, store carefully, and replenish as needed.

Spices:          allspice, anise seeds, asafoetida (hing), celery seed, cinnamon, coriander, clove, cumin, ginger, Kapha Churna nutmeg, mustard seeds, turmeric

Herbs:          basil, dill, fennel, oregano, parsley,thyme, rosemary, sage, saffron, savory, tarragon

Grains & Others:   barley, barley flour, cornmeal, millet, rice, rice cakes, honey, walnuts, lentils, ghee, corn oil, herbal teas, black tea, and coffee

## Sparking Kapha's Digestion

Kapha usually appreciates a pungent appetizer to start the meal. Grated fresh ginger with a spritz of lemon juice makes a simple condiment. Or even a pinch of powdered ginger under the tongue just before eating will spark Kapha's appetite. A steaming bowl of peppery soup, a teaspoon or two of rice and ghee, or pungent little condiments will help ignite the digestive fires and make a meal most useful for Kapha. Because agni is so variable in Kapha's digestion, pungent tastes should be interspersed throughout the meal. This is especially true when serving foods that are heavy and more difficult to digest.

## About the Recipes

Although the recipes and sample menu in this chapter are especially good for maintaining Kapha in balance, many of these recipes can be prepared for a meal to serve to people with different dietary needs.

Many times a recipe that is good for balancing one body type is also good for one of the others. When using AyurVedic menu planning principles, it is difficult to create recipes exclusively for one constitution because so many foods are good for everyone.

When you're planning a family meal that includes a variety of dishes, remember that each person will simply select the amount from each dish that is best for him. Because some of these recipes are useful for more than the Kapha constitution, they may appear—sometimes with minor changes—in the Pitta or Vata sections of this book as well. All the recipes appealing throughout this book are collected in Chapter 10, "An AyurVeda Recipe Companion."

## An AyurVedic meal has:

- foods with all six tastes and qualities
- variety of colors, textures, and flavors to stimulate the eye and palate
- thoughtful order of presentation starting with a pungent appetizer,
- alternating light and heavy courses,
- ends with a light sweet.

## Sample Kapha Menu

GOLDEN YUMMIES
(Sweet, Oily, Slightly Pungent)

VEGETABLE SOUP WITH FRESH HERBS
( Pungent, Light )

VEGETABLE BARLEY SAUTE
( Sweet, Astringent, Light, Oily )
or
ROASTED AND SPICED BARLEY
(Pungent, Sweet, Astringent, Oily, Light )

TOSSED GREEN SALAD with VINAIGRETTE
(Pungent, Bitter, Astringent , Oily )

CORNBREAD AND BUTTER
(Sweet, Salty, Hot, Light )

FRESH GINGER COOKIES
(Sweet, Pungent, Salty, Dry)

WHITE FIGS a la KAPHA
(Sweet, Heavy)

## Golden Yummies

These delicious little appetizers are sweet, oily, and a little pungent. They are good for all doshas when served as hot hors d'oeuvres. Allow 2 to 3 per person. The topping is good by itself as a sweet condiment or chutney.

Makes 2 cups

For the Topping:

> 1 1/2 tablespoons ghee
> 1/2 teaspoon cayenne
> 1/3 cup milk or cream
> 1 to 2 tablespoons sugar, to taste
> 1/8 teaspoon allspice
> 1/8 to 1/4 teaspoon saffron, crushed
> 1/4 cup raisins
> 1 to 1 1/2 cups coconut—finely chopped is best, but flaked will do

In a small saucepan or frying pan, heat ghee over moderately high flame. Then add cayenne and stir about one minute. Add milk, sugar, allspice, and crumbled saffron threads. Bring to a boil, stirring often. Milk should begin turning golden yellow. Reduce heat to simmer. Stir in raisins and 1 cup coconut. Beat well as the mixture leaves sides of the pan. If it is too liquid, add more coconut, a tablespoon at a time, until the mixture is just moist but not wet. Set aside until ready to assemble, or serve as a chutney.

To Assemble:

> 1/2 tablespoon ghee
> 1/8 teaspoon cayenne
> 1/8 teaspoon ground ginger
> Cashew, almond, or sesame nut butter
> Wheat or other mild flavored crackers

Heat the ghee, cayenne, and ginger in a small pan. Add 2 or 3 tablespoons of topping per person. Fry over high heat, stirring until heated thoroughly. Spread each cracker with 1/2 teaspoon nut butter, then top with one teaspoon hot coconut mixture. Serve warm. If prepared in advance, put under broiler for 30 seconds before serving.

## Vegetable Soup with Fresh Herbs

This light and pungent soup is excellent for Kapha. Its basis is Kapha Broth Variations on this soup can be made by selecting three or more Kapha-reducing seasonal vegetables for the broth and adding Kapha appropriate herbs. Semolina pasta or rice make it a little thicker, but they can be eliminated or cooked barley can be substituted by those following a very light diet. It increases Pitta and Vata slightly.

Serves 6 to 8

2 quarts water
2 teaspoons salt
1 teaspoon coarsely ground pepper
4 cups cauliflower in bite-size pieces
1 large carrot, sliced
1 cup green beans cut in 1-inch pieces
1/4 cup parsley, chopped
1 teaspoon French tarragon, minced, or 1/2 teaspoon dried tarragon
1 to 2 teaspoons minced lemon basil or lemon thyme,
   or 1 teaspoon dried thyme leaves
3/4 cup tiny semolina pasta or rice

Bring water to a boil. Add salt, pepper, and vegetables. Cover and bring just to a boil. Lower to simmer and sprinkle chopped herbs on top. Stir once, gently. Cover and turn off heat and do not lift lid for 20 to 30 minutes.

When ready to serve, bring pot to a boil and add tiny semolina pasta or rice. Simmer for 8 to 10 minutes and serve.

## Vegetable Barley Sauté

A light, easily digested main dish that is just right for Kapha, but can be eaten by anyone as part of a balanced meal. This recipe adds sweet, astringent tastes and light and oily qualities. The use of sprouted urad beans—whole black gram—adds a sweet, nutty flavor. These sprouts are very nourishing and somewhat weight producing. For those who want to use this dish for dieting, mung bean or brown lentil sprouts can be used instead of the more fattening urad.

Serves 4

Prepare Barley:

> 2 1/4 cups water
> 2/3 cup barley, pearled or unhulled
> 1/2 teaspoon salt
> 2 teaspoon olive oil

In a heavy 1-quart pan boil the water, Add salt and rinsed barley. Cover and simmer gently for 40 minutes until the barley is soft but is still holding its shape. When cooked, toss with olive oil, cover, and set aside until ready to serve.

Prepare the vegetables:

> 2 teaspoons sesame oil
> 2 tablespoons sunflower seeds
> 1/2 teaspoon salt
> 1/2 teaspoon coarsely ground pepper
> 1/2 cup shredded zucchini
> 3/4 cup shredded carrots
> 1/2 cup minced celery
> 1 cup urad beans, sprouted

Heat sesame oil in large wok or large heavy frying pan over medium high heat. Add sunflower seeds, salt and pepper and sauté about one minute or until seeds are just browning. Add zucchini and carrots and toss with seeds, fying for about a minute. Then add minced celery and sprouts and cook another minute. Turn off heat, cover until ready to serve.

continues

## Vegetable Barley Sauté continued

Just before serving:

      1/2 teaspoon olive oil
      1 teaspoon crushed sage
      1 teaspoon fresh thyme, minced
          or
       1/2 teaspoon dried thyme, crushed
      Lemon wedges

In a heavy frying pan heat 1/2 teaspoon olive oil. Add cooked barley, sage, and thyme, mixing well and heat thoroughly. Mound on a serving plate with an indentation in the center. Pile the sautéed vegetables on top. Decorate with lemon wedges.

## To Sprout Whole Beans

Use whole lentil beans (gram) when sprouting. Use 1/2 cup washed lentils. Place them in a covered bowl or jar, set in a warm place, and rinse in tepid water 3 or 4 times a day. They are ready to use when just slightly sprouted in about 24 hours.

## Vegtables with Spiced and Roasted Barley

Everyone can eat some of this dish as part of a balanced meal, but for Kapha it is a first choice as a main dish because the barley is essentially light in quality, easily digested, and not filling. The outstanding tastes of this recipe are pungent, sweet, and salty.

Serves 6 to 8

To prepare the barley:

3 tablespoons ghee
1/2 teaspoon cayenne
1 cup barley, rinsed
1 1/2 teaspoons salt
3 1/2 cups hot water

Heat ghee in a heavy skillet or 2-quart pot over moderate heat. Stir in the cayenne. After one minute stir in barley. Roast barley by continuously stirring until grains are medium brown. Watch carefully not to burn it. Then sprinkle on salt, add hot water, and stir once or twice. Cover tightly and simmer for about 1 hour. It's all right if some liquid remains. Fluff up and set aside while you prepare vegetables. Or make ahead and prepare vegetables just before serving.

To prepare the vegetables:

1 cup broccoli, cut in flowerets
2 tablespoons olive oil
1 teaspoon minced fresh ginger or 1/2 teaspoon ground ginger
1/4 cup sesame seeds
1/4 cup roasted pumpkin seeds
1 sweet red pepper, cut in 1-inch squares
1 cup Swiss chard (mixed ruby and white look best)—washed and chopped
1/2 cup beet green, washed and chopped
2 teaspoons salt
1/2 teaspoon coarsely ground pepper

Steam broccoli for 3 to 4 minutes and set aside.

continues

## Vegtables with Spiced and Roasted Barley, continued

Heat the oil in a wok or large heavy frying pan. Add ginger and sesame seeds. Fry over moderate heat until seeds start to pop. Add half the pumpkin seeds, stir, add red peppers, stir; and add chard and beet greens. Add steamed broccoli, salt, and pepper. Toss well and cover. Turn off heat and let vegetables steam while you reheat the barley over medium heat until any remaining liquid is gone. Stir in remaining 1/4 cup pumpkin seeds and spread the barley on serving platter.

Arrange the vegetables on the bed of barley and serve.

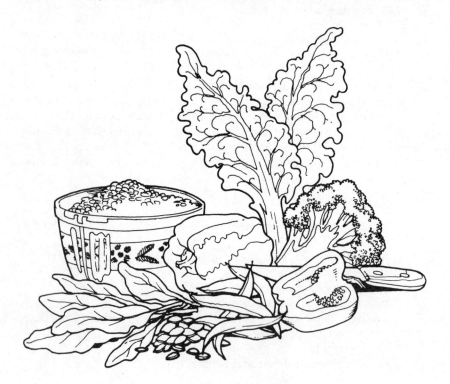

## Tossed Green Salad

A tossed green salad of several types of lettuce and other fresh greens adds texture and color to a meal. It also contributes some of the bitter, astringent, and pungent tastes we want in a balanced menu. By adding touches of such fresh herbs as chopped French tarragon, basil (especially tassty are cinnamon, anise, and lemon basil leaves), chopped parsley, or cilantro, you'll enjoy pleasant little surprises in your salad.

Greens should be torn into bite-size pieces. You shouldn't be forced to chop through a tossed salad with a knife, or have to eat large lettuce leaves whole. Allow about one loosely packed quart of greens for every 2 people. It is best to dress a salad just before it is eaten. Any greens that have been dressed with oil should not be saved.

Tossed green salads are especialy good for Kapha to eat every day. A pleasant subtle dressing for Kapha is a squeeze of lemon or orange juice, or a simple vinaigrette. All salad dressings in this book have been rated good for all types when mixed well and combined with a green salad. For a Kapha menu choose any of these.

## Simple Vinaigrette Dressing

1/4 cup oil
1 tablespoon warm water
1 tablespoon vinegar
1/4 teaspoon salt

Place all ingredients in a small jar, cover tightly, and shake vigorously.

## Cornbread

Cornbread is a sweet, salty, hot, light bread that is good for both Kapha and those wanting to reduce weight. As with many other Kapha-reducing foods, cornbread is good to eat during a light fast, or as part of a light evening meal. Those wanting to lose weight can skip the additional butter or use very little.

Serves 6 to 8

    1 cup white flour
    1 cup cornmeal
    5 teaspoons baking powder
    3/4 teaspoon salt
    1 cup milk
    2 tablespoons butter or ghee
    4 tablespoons sugar

Preheat oven to 375°.

Sift all dry ingredients together except sugar. Heat milk, ghee or butter, and sugar in a saucepan and stir until sugar is dissolved. Then stir into mixed dry ingredients until just moistened. Batter will be thick and a little lumpy. Spread batter in a oiled 9-inch pan and bake for 30 to 35 minutes until light brown.

## Fresh Ginger Cookies

This cookie is one of those rare desserts that Kapha can eat in more than small amounts. They are sweet, pungent, salty, and astringent. Since they are made entirely with barley flour, one of Kapha's best grains, and contain a generaous amount of ginger, they are a good dessert to serve to weight watchers. The fresh ginger really make these sparkle! These cookies also travel well for sending as gifts.

Makes about 2 dozen

> 4 cups barley flour
> 2 teaspoons baking soda
> 1/4 teaspoon salt
> 1 tablespoon cinnamon
> 1/2 teaspoon cloves
> 1/2 cup oil or ghee
> 1 1/3 cups molasses
> 3 tablespoons fresh ginger, finely grated
> or
> 1 tablespoon ground ginger

Preheat oven to 350°.

Mix all ingredients together and roll into 1-inch balls. Bake on a lightly greased cookie sheet for about 15 minutes or until light brown. The centers will be soft. Cool on a rack and store securely.

## White Figs a la Kapha

Although other figs like black or Mission figs are nourishing, none is held in such esteem as Calmyrnas—known in AyurVeda as *anjier*. They are sold dried at most supermarkets and health food stores.

Plump some white Calmyrna figs in a vegetable steamer for 5 minutes. Serve warm. One or two figs and a few fresh ginger cookies make a good dessert for Kapha.

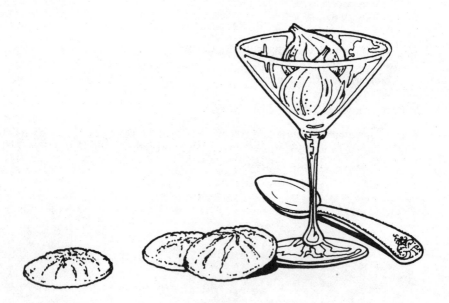

## Other Recipes Especially for Kapha

When planning your own menus, try any of these recipes appropriate for a Kapha-balancing diet. They can be found in Chapter 10, "An AyurVeda Recipe Companion." Some of the recipes may also appear in Pitta Vand Vata chapters or elsewhere in this book with minor variations.

## Beverages

Bed and Breakfast Drink
Fragrantly Spiced Lassi
Indian Spicy Milk Tea
Plain Lassi
Saffron Milk Tea
Three-in-One Samhita Supreme II

## Appetizers

Cheese Crackers
Golden Panir Cubes
Curried Herb Cheese Dip
Pineapple-Ginger Cream Spread

## Salads

Confetti Rice Salad
Macedonia di Frutta
Tossed Green Salad

## Dressings, Sauces, Spreads, and Marinades

Simple Vinaigrette Dressing
Herbed Vinaigrette
Deanna's Vinaigrette
Scrumptious Sesame Orange Dressing and Sauce
Pitta Churna Salad Dressing and Marinade
Raspberry Vinaigrette
Ginger Soy Gravy
Cream Tahini Sauce

## Other Basics

Ghee
Panir and Ricotta Soft Cheese
Sprouting Whole Beans and Seeds
Kapha Broth

## Breads

French Bread
Little Flat Breads
Puris and Chapatis
Squash Rolls

## Soups

Ginger Carrot Soup
Potage Printanier

## Main Dishes

BakedWild Rice Casserole
Curried Vegetables and Panir
Fagioloni in Umido Volponi
Green and Gold Squash
Layered Vegetable Loaf

## Side Dishes (as part of a main meal)

Couscous
Fried-Spiced Potatoes
Moroccan Delight
Petit Pois Laitue
Saffron Rice
Simple Rice Pilaf
Sweet Summer Curry

## Desserts

Apple Pie without Sugar
Fruit Shortcake
Ginger Spice Cake with Lemon Sauce
Italian Hazelnut Cookies
Jam Diagonals
Lemon Scones
Lemony Date Bars
Marble Crumb Cake
Plain Shortbread
Super Chocolate Brownies
Sweet Fruit and Spice Bread
Toasty Cinnamon Bar Cookies

## For A Kapha-Balancing Diet

### FAVOR

General:      Lighter Diet, Dry Foods, Warm Foods and Drinks,
              Pungent, Bitter, and Astringent Tastes
Dairy:        Low-Fat Milk or moderate amounts of Whole Milk
Sweetener:    Honey, in moderation
Grains:       Barley, Corn, Millet, Buckwheat, Rye
Fruits:       Apple, Pomegranate, Persimmon, Papaya, Watermelon
Vegetables:   Asparagus, Eggplant, Beets, Broccoli, Potato, Cabbage,
              Carrot, Cauliflower, Celery, Green Leafy Vegetables,
              Sprouts, Radish, Hot Peppers, Squash, Zucchini
Spices:       Most Spices (see Ingredients Charts)
Nuts:         Walnuts, Blanched Almonds--small amounts
Beans:        Most Lentils
Beverages:    Warm Water, Most Herbal Teas, Coffee,  Black Tea,
              Some Fruit Juices (in moderation), Vegetable Juices
Animal Food For Non-Vegetarians:  Chicken, Turkey

### REDUCE

General:      Large quantities of Food; Unctuous, Heavy, Cold Food and
              Drinks, Sweet, Sour, and Salty Tastes
Dairy:        Yogurt, Cream, Butter, Sour Cream, Cheese,Whole Milk
              and Ghee (in large amounts)
Sweeteners:   Sugar-Cane Products, Molasses
Oils:         All except small amounts of Almond, Corn, Walnut,
              Sunflower, or Sesame oils
Grains:       Large quantities of Wheat, Rice, or Oats
Fruits:       Grapes, Melons, Avocado, Coconut, Dried Fruit, Banana,
              Orange, Pineapple, Plums, Berries
Vegetables:   Tomato, Cucumber, Sweet Potato, Sweet Peppers
Beans:        Beans, Tofu and other Soy Products,
Spices:       Caraway, Cardamom, Poppyseeds, Garlic, Salt
Nuts:         All  except Walnuts, small amounts Blanched Almonds
Beverages:    Iced /Cold Drinks, Cold Milk, Milkshakes, Buttermilk,
              Lassi, Sweet Fruit Juices
Animal Foods For Non-Vegetarians:  Seafood, Beef, Pork

# Chapter 5

# *Planning Good Meals*

## Menu Planning

Successful AyurVedic cooking is a matter of knowing how food influences each of the different body types throughout the year and then planning well-balanced meals accordingly. All of the sample menus and recipes in this book have been developed and rated by experts in AyurVeda for their specific action on each body type. These are offered as examples for you as you adapt your favorite recipes and create your own balanced recipes and meals. Undertake AyurVedic menu planning with variety in mind. Even those menus specifically designed for Vata, Pitta, or Kapha contain a wide enough range of tastes and qualities so anyone can choose from them and feel satisfied.

*Proper diet is considered as the Self.*

- The Upanishads

## The Varied Menu

When planning and preparing a full dinner menu, especially for family members or friends with all types of dietary needs, the universal principal of "the whole is more than the sum of the parts" should be your guide. All the various herbs and spices, vegetables, fruits, grains, and cooking techniques combine to make a finished recipe with an overall effect that is greater than that of any single ingredient or preparation method. And the combination of four or five dishes served at a meal interact to produce an effect that is greater than that of any single dish. Usually the ingredient used in the greatest amount has a dominant influence in a recipe.

Different cooking processes--frying or roasting compared with boiling or steaming--may change the predicted quality of an individual ingredient or the whole recipe. Boiling or steaming a potato makes it moist and somewhat lighter in quality, deep frying produces a heavier, oily potato, and dry roasting makes the potato light and dry. But the effect of the taste in the menu does not change with the cooking technique--pungent remains pungent and sweet stays sweet, no matter how the ingredient is prepared.

Whenever possible use more than one method of heating/cooking in each main meal. An all-boiled meal can seem rather bland or uninteresting, and a meal where everything is stir-fried and deep fried is heavy to digest. Varied menus are interesting, balanced, and satisfying for everyone. Sumptuous menus with delicious food is a goal of AyurVedic cooking.

91

# Points To Remember
# When Planning A Meal

- Meals Look Colorful
  Smell Delicious
  Taste Wonderful

- Choose Ingredients
  Appropriate to the Season
  Fresh as Possible

- Include Six Tastes
  Six Qualities
  Three Categories

- Always Follow Seasonal Considerations
  Dictates of the Body's Needs
  Common Sense

## Tastes, Qualities, Groups

No matter who you are cooking for always be sure each main meal has some sweet, salty, sour, bitter, astringent, and pungent tastes. Include some of each of the six qualities, hot/cold, dry/oily, heavy/light, as well. A large proportion of any menu comes from the Superior (*sattva* ) category or group, less from the Active (*rajas* ), and a tiny bit from the Dull (*tamas* ) group.

Just as eating only one or two taste and quality combinations leads to imbalance, in the AyurVedic view exclusively eating food with superior or sattvic effects (as salutary as they are) would not represent all the balance found in nature. The human body is seen as a small, complete version of the universe in which every element in creation can be found. Even though the very active and dull categories of food aren't as healthful when eaten in anything other than moderate to tiny amounts, AyurVeda recommends they be represented in the healthfully balanced diet. The following chart gives examples of the three categories, known as *gunas* in Sanskrit, and how they relate to diet.

*Food
has a very great influence on the mind because
everything we eat and drink is transported by
the blood which sustains the nervous system.
Therefore the quality of the food
has a great deal to do
with the quality of the
mind.*

- Maharishi Mahesh Yogi

# The Three Categories of Diet

| Superior<br>(*Sattva*) | Active<br>(*Rajas*) | Dull<br>(*Tamas*) |
|---|---|---|
| Diet which develops mental and physical strength, longevity, health, creates happiness and love. Filled with Rasayana value for mind, body, and nature.<br><br>Qualities: sweet, light, oily, contains all 6 tastes, balanced protein, vitamins, and nutrients. | If eaten in excess creates burning feeling, unhappiness, anger, discomfort, or disease<br><br>Qualities: dry, hot, sour, salty. | More than a small amount in diet will create dull, listless mind and behavior, and serious illness.<br><br>Qualities: *extremely* cold, hot, heavy, dry, or sour. Spoiled, stale/left-over, burned food. |

| Favor | Reduce | Avoid |
|---|---|---|
| Cow's milk, buttermilk, ghee, sweet fruits and juices.<br><br>Mung beans and lentils, wheat, rice. Fresh whole food. | Very pungent, sour, salty, or dry vegetables and spices. Too much hing, black pepper, vinegar, tofu, peanuts, chicken, meat, fish, cheese. Canned, frozen, or bottled foods. | Extremely hot, sour, pungent tastes. Cooked food sitting out many hours. Cold and dry, tasteless, burned, spoiled, dirty food. Food already tasted by others.<br><br>Onions, mushrooms, garlic, wine.<br>*Large amounts* of meat, fish, chicken, cayenne peppers, other chilis. |

Every meal contains something from each category. Most of the diet is from the Superior category, a small part is Active, and a tiny bit is Dull.

## Menu Planning by the Season

The weather and the seasons have their own predictable influences on our health.  Knowing this, one of the best things anyone can do to prevent illness is to eat foods that tend to maintain doshic balance during seasonal changes while nourishing the body at its most fundamental level.  In seasonal cooking it is most important to follow the principle of similarities and differences as described in Chapter 1.  During the season or in the weather most like your dominant dosha, eating foods that have qualities like the weather aggravates that dosha and sends the system out of balance. It can take a month or two, or sometimes until the next season, before the accumulated imbalance shows up as illness.

## Seasons and Weather Affect the Doshas

| Season | Dosha | Weather |
|---|---|---|
| Late Autumn / Winter | Vata | Increases in cold, dry, windy weather |
| Spring | Kapha | Increases in humid, heavy, wet, cold weather |
| Summer /Early Autumn | Pitta | Increases in sunny, dry, hot weather |

# 5  The AyurVeda Cookbook

## Guide for Menu Planning by Constitution and Season

| Constitution | Winter | Summer/Fall | Spring |
|---|---|---|---|
| Vata | V | V | V |
| Pitta | P | P | P |
| Kapha | K | K | K |
| Vata-Pitta/Pitta-Vata | V | P | V |
| Vata-Kapha/Kapha-Vata | K | V | V (if thin) |
| Pitta-Kapha/Kapha-Pitta | K | P | P/K K (if heavy) |
| Vata-Pitta- and Kapha | K | P | V |

V= vata-balancing diet, P= pitta-balancing diet, K= kapha-balancing diet.

## Menu Planning by Constitution and Season

The chapters in this book that are written specially for each body type further describe the influences of the seasons and seasonal cooking.

In reading the following chart notice that during the weather and season most like your nature it's best to eat meals that balance your dominant dosha(s). Very thin people with Vata-Kapha constitutions follow a Vata-decreasing diet year round rather than lose weight on a Kapha-reducing diet. Those Kapha-Pitta or Pitta-Kapha types who need to lose weight maintain a "very tender balance" by continuing to follow a Kapha-decreasing diet even in summer, but adding cooling fruits and other foods, too.

# A Week's Meals At A Glance

| Day | Menu |
|---|---|
| 1 | Vegetable Soup with Herbs, Stuffed Pasta Shells, Tossed Salad, Italian Bread, Strawberry-Yogurt Pie. |
| 2 | Curried Herb Dip and Chips, Tofu Nut Patties, Mashed Potatoes/ Ginger Soy Gravy, Steamed Mixed Vegetables, Coleslaw, Tossed Salad, Ginger Spice Cake with Lemon Sauce. |
| 3 | Cheese Crackers, Baked Lentil Soup, Green & Gold Squash, Baked Wild Rice Casserole, Stewed Apples, Swedish Chocolate Cream Pie. |
| 4 | Ginger Carrot Soup, Baked Potatoes with Various Fillings, Steamed Cabbage with Hot Caraway Dressing, Squash Rolls, Tossed Salad, White Figs in Apricot Cream, Cookies. |
| 5 | Sliced Fresh Ginger, Zucchini-Tomato Fry, Barley or Couscous, Stuffed Artichokes, Tossed Salad and Pitta Dressing, Old Fashioned Cake. |
| 6 | Dahl and Saffron Rice, Curried Vegetables and Panir, Puris, Condiments, Raita, Almond Custard Fresh Fruit Pie. |
| 7 | Rest Day: Light Meal, French Potato Soup, Steamed Vegetable or Cornbread, warm Herbal Tea. |

An AyurVedic weekly menu for main meals might look like this. The recipes can be found in Chapter 10 "The AyurVeda Recipe Companion." You can easily adapt your own favorite recipes by following basic Ayur-Vedic guidelines. Light meals and foods for fasting are discussed in Chapter 9.

## Serving Large Groups

Serving a great variety of foods, with many condiments in small decorative bowls, buffet style, is an easy solution to large group needs for variety and balance. Each person can select greater amounts of the foods most nourishing for him and less of those that he simply needs to nibble on for overall balance. Preparing simple entrees or side dishes accompanied by a variety of toppings or sauces is not only easy on the cook, but abundant choices give a feeling of opulence, making even simple meals festive for everyone. Serving baked potatoes and halves of baked squash served with ghee or butter, a broccoli cream sauce, sour cream mixed with Mexican picanté sauce, curried vegetables, spicy dahl, and other pungent-tasting toppings (to aid digestion) will give everyone plenty to choose from.

## Some Basic Condiments

One way to keep menu planning simple but still produce interesting meals is to maintain certain family favorites and seasonal standards like rice and other grains, lentils, potatoes, pasta, mixed steamed vegetables, tofu, and so forth all year round but prepare sauces, condiments, dressings, and marinades that highlight the particular tastes and qualities you want. These are a few condiments for daily meals.

| | |
|---|---|
| Chopped Nuts | plain walnut pieces, pecans or other nuts or cashews and blanched slivered almonds fried in a little ghee |
| Coconut | flaked or shredded—plain or lightly roasted in heavy pan |
| Pickles | Sweet or gherkins to stimulate appetite |
| Citrus Fruits | lemon, lime, and orange wedges |
| Fresh Ginger | chopped or thinly peeled, and served plain or marinated in lemon juice and salt |

*When dining out be aware of what is best for you to eat, what you feel like eating, and order accordingly.*

## Balanced Meals for Children

When cooking for children the same AyurVedic guidelines for balance apply. Give children more of what they should have and less of what causes imbalances. If children resist certain tastes and qualities or have not yet developed a liking for them, then include small amounts of that taste in something they enjoy. It is just as important to plan balanced menus for children as for adults; their recipes may require more clever adjustments. It is one of the age-old challenges of parenthood.

*As you eat so shall you think.*

- Dr. P.D. Subhedar

## Recipe Design

When creating a new recipe first consider the action of each ingredient. Later, when planning the complete menu, see how each finished recipe interacts with all the others in the menu to make a meal balanced in tastes and qualities. This is not as difficult as it may sound. We know the influences of many of the ingredients commonly used in American cooking. Many are listed in the Ingredients Charts which may serve as a starting point and general guide for the design and adaptation of your own recipes When planning, however, keep in mind that when these ingredients are combined in a recipe and heated, the result is sometimes changed slightly in the cooking process—boiling liquids and frying grains in a small amount of oil lightens them, while the deep-frying process or using unsaturated oils make light foods heavier in quality. When several dishes containing widely differing tastes and qualities are served at the same meal, there will be a re-balancing of the overall effect within the entire menu. With the addition of each dish featuring another group of tastes and qualities, the entire meal becomes more varied and suitable for many different people to eat. So one recipe has its own part to play in the whole meal but, unless it contains some overpowering taste or quality, it is only one of the players and not the prima donna.

## Healthy Combinations of Tastes and Qualities

AyurVeda has identified how the different tastes and qualities when combined give the most healthful results. It considers certain ingredients as superior, good, and inferior when combined. Inferior combinations may or may not taste unpleasant, but the results usually lead to lack of balance in the doshas or illness.

Many superior food combinations are a standard part of the American cuisine, but it might be of interest to know why certain combinations are good for us. For instance, is a mixed green salad with vinaigrette dressing healthful? Astringent, bitter, pungent, sweet, light, and dry properties all work well together (see the following chart). You might think of them as friends who have good influences on one another. These are the tastes and qualities in a typical tossed salad with simple dressing. The greens in a salad (more than pale iceberg lettuce, please) are light in quality, and sweet, bitter, astringent, and a little pungent in tastes. By adding such chopped fresh herbs as, parsley (pungent, astringent, slightly bitter), basil (pungent), tarragon (pungent, bitter), or thyme (pungent, astringent, bitter), the variety of qualities and the depth of taste increases. And then, when all of these are tossed with an oil and vinegar dressing, the salad is a further blending of dry and light qualities with astringent and sweet tastes that work nicely together.

This combination is not only full of the tastes and qualities most beneficial to Kapha types, but it is healthful for everyone when served as part of a complete meal. Combinations of bitter, pungent, and astringent tastes are often lacking in American main dishes. By including a tossed salad in the dinner menu the whole meal is easily balanced. And best of all, by using this concept of combining the best tastes and qualities, meals will not be a haphazard result of putting things together in hopes of making "creative" meals. As an Ayurvedic cook you *know* the healthful benefits of everything you serve.

*Anything in the world is good
if taken in the proper quantity—
in balance.*

- Dr. P. D. Subhedar

# How Ingredients Combine

| Quality | Taste | | |
|---------|-------|---|---|
|  | Superior | Good | Inferior |
| Heavy | Sweet | Astringent | Salty |
| Light | Bitter | Pungent | Sour |
| Dry | Astringent | Sour | Salty |
| Oily | Sweet | Pungent | Bitter |
| Hot | Salty | Sour | Pungent |
| Cold | Sweet | Astringent | Bitter |

## Designing a New Recipe: An Example

One way to design a new recipe is to begin by thinking of the kind of dish you want to make combining all "superior" and "good" tastes and qualities that appeal to you. This is how the recipe for the appetizer "Golden Yummies" came about. These are small crackers topped with a brilliant gold, warm mixture of coconut, raisins, spices, and cashew butter. An excellent appetizer will be sweet, rather pungent, oily, heavy, and colorful, or any combination of these. The most stimulating and appetizing colors are red, gold-orange, and yellow.

The ingredients in "Golden Yummies" repeat all these properties.

| | | | |
|---|---|---|---|
| Ghee | sweet, oily, cold | Sugar | sweet, heavy, cold |
| Cayenne | pungent, dry, light | Raisins | sweet, heavy |
| Saffron | sweet, pungent, oily | Cream | sweet, oily, heavy, cold |
| Allspice | pungent, astringent | Cashew butter | sweet, heavy, oily |
| Coconut | sweet, heavy,oily | | |

By looking at the Taste and Quality Combinations chart, we see that the heavy and oily qualities in the coconut, cashew butter, and cream combine in a superior way with sweet tasting ghee, saffron, coconut, sugar, cream, raisins,and cashew butter.  In the art of recipe design this is a larger than average number of ingredients in the superior range, where even two or three superior combinations are fine.  The pungent aspects of a good appetizer that help to heat the palate or the digestion are well-represented in this recipe by cayenne, saffron, and allspice.  Had similar but bitter-tasting ingredients such as turmeric and poppy seeds been used for color instead of saffron, the recipe would not have had its superior effect and would not have been as healthful.  Everyone can eat a few Golden Yummies before a meal.  It is especially appetizing for Vata and Kapha.

*Diet is not for filling the stomach cavity*
*Diet is for yagya.*
*Offer food to others and take the*
*rest for yourself.*

- Dr. H.S. Kasture

## "Companion" Cooking

Another way of looking at combining foods and ingredients is to compare it to a popular gardening term, "companion gardening," in which certain plants are thought to grow better near other plants. In AvurVedic cooking knowing what likes (and does not like) to be with what makes recipe design easy.

Cinnamon likes Chocolate,

Vanilla prefers warm, sweet liquids and cakes.

Milk and Cream do not like lemon, salt, or fish,

But Milk loves Butter, Ghee, and Nutmeg.

Nutmeg likes Spinach and Zucchini, too.

Ghee likes some spices better than others:

Cumin, Fenugreek, Hing, Coriander, and Turmeric,

to name a few.

# 5  The AyurVeda Cookbook

*Chapter 6*

*Something for Everyone*

## Eat What You Like

From what you've read thus far it may seem that AyurVedic cooking is limited to the single person with very specific needs. But those who cook for families or groups needn't worry. One of AyurVeda's strengths is that not only is the effect of every ingredient known and predictable for each person, but a great many foods are good for everyone to eat.[1] Most of these fall into in the "superior" category of nourishing foods that were presented in Chapter 5.

Eat the foods you enjoy. It's good to remember that by eating too much of a limited variety of foods, even of the universally good foods discussed in this chapter, Vata, Pitta, and Kapha are inclined to increase or otherwise gradually become out of balance. Moderation is always the key to healthy eating. But that consideration aside, what foods *can* all of us enjoy?

## Water

Many people don't think of water as "food." But water is essential to everyone's diet and good digestion. Uncarbonated spring water is fine to drink and tap water, too, in areas with good water quality. When there is a choice, the best temperature for drinking water is tepid or warm in winter and on cool days, and cool or tepid in the summer or on hot days.

*AyurVeda declares water to be the first choice among all drinks.*

To heat water, bring it to a full boil and then let it cool until it is a comfortable drinking temperature. Boiled water is thought to be better for the body because of the molecular changes that occur, making it lighter and easier to digest for those people with Kapha constitutions, who need lighter qualities in their diets. Vata always appreciates drinking warm water.

Ice-cold water is not beneficial, even in the heat of summer, although people with Pitta constitutions can drink refrigerated or chilled drinks during hot weather. For good digestion and lasting refreshment drinks made with lots of ice are not recommended, even for Pitta types.

## Water with Meals

Water is the best drink to serve at all meals. It should be sipped with the entire meal that is, before eating, during the meal, between courses, when not chewing food, and after eating. You might think of it as "layering" the food with liquid. But remember, only fill the stomach to two-thirds of its capacity, so that at the end of the meal one-third of the stomach contains food and one-third water. The rest should be left empty to allow for the activity of comfortable digestion.

## Juices or Teas: Before and After Eating

Fruit juices and other drinks are best appreciated by themselves or with a light snack, rather than as a part of the meal. Exceptions are juices that are served as appetizers. A small glass of apple juice or pomegranate juice can be served as an appetizer for everyone before a meal. Pomegranate juice, a highly recommended appetizer, should be served at room temperature or only slightly chilled. It is sold in quart bottles at most health food stores.

Some people may prefer to end a meal with a warm cup of herbal tea, especially in winter. Tea should be served 10 or 15 minutes after the meal is finished, not as an on-going part of the meal. The Ingredients Chart in the Appendix lists specific teas that have been tested for their effects on each constitutional type.

In warm weather a glass of lassi makes a refreshing ending to a main meal.

## Coffee and Black Tea

Of the great variety of teas and coffees to choose from, black teas and limited amounts of coffee are all right for Kapha to drink, and to a lesser extent, those with Pitta constitutions, if it is comfortable. Whichever of the many different flavors of coffee or tea is your favorite, or whether it is decaffeinated or not, the effect is the same because the bitter taste dominates all of them. The bitter taste increases Vata.

## More About Herbal Teas

While investigating teas, the AyurVedic research team sampled all the herbal tea blends from Celestial Seasonings, one of the most widely available brands. Most of these were blends of certain herbs and spices with a predominating rosehip/hibiscus base that decreased Vata, increased Pitta and Kapha.

Two appetizing blends, however, were considered most useful for their tonic or healthful effects. "Pelican Punch," judged good for all doshas with its sweet, astringent, slightly bitter tastes, is stimulating, sharp, and a good appetizer. The second, "Emperor's Choice," is also sweet, astringent, and a little bitter. Ginseng and other herbs make it a good tonic that increases appetite but not weight. This blend is especially good for Kapha body types and those wishing to lose weight. Both teas can be served as appetizers before meals or by themselves. One would not end a meal with these teas.

By using one or a combination of herbs or spices listed in the Ingredients Charts you can make your own simple herbal teas that appeal to your tastes and dietary needs. Or serve AyurVedic teas especially formulated to benefit each body type during the changing seasons. If not available at your grocery or health food store,these teas can be ordered from Maharishi Ayur-Veda Products Corporation.[2]

*AyurVeda is dedicated to all those who want to become good eaters.*

\- Dr. H. S. Kasture

## A Good AyurVedic Principle for Everyone

By now you know that certain foods and spices may increase or reduce the balance of Vata, Pitta, or Kapha in your physiology. But what if you're particularly fond of something that you know will aggravate your doshas—do you need to eliminate it altogether? Not necessarily; just reduce the quantity.

The AyurVedic principle of moderation, applied to all foods, is the best to follow. For instance, you may wish to have a cup of chamomile tea and you notice on the Ingredients Chart that this herb increases Vata, decreases Kapha, and has a neutral effect on Pitta when drunk in moderation. If you are Vata type who loves chamomile tea, then once or twice a week enjoy a small amount of it. If is is a windy, cold day another Vata-decreasing tea would have a better result. This is an example of moderation in AyurVeda. Drinking chamomile tea every day or several times a day is excessive for Vata, and even Pitta, to some extent. The situation is the same for Vata types drinking coffee or black tea. Moderation gives the most comfort in the long run.

Similarly, fresh ginger tea is a marvelously refreshing and stimulating drink for both Vata and Kapha types; but even those with a Pitta constitution may have some on a cool day or during the cold season, if they want it. Pungent teas are entirely too stimulating for those with Pitta constitutions in warm or hot weather.

Remember, too, in AyurVedic cooking just a pinch of some spice can change the effect of a recipe. It is not necessary to use great quantities of herbs and spices to achieve a balance of tastes. It's just a matter of using common sense when applying the information in the Ingredients Charts and also trying to satisfy your appetite at the same time.

## Milk: Nature's Most Perfect Food

Sweet-tasting, heavy, and nourishing milk is nature's most perfect food. Of the several kinds of milk, cow's milk is most nutritious for everyone at every age. Whenever possible heat milk and serve it warm. Just bring it to a boil and allow to cool to a comfortable drinking temperature. As with water, this process of heating makes milk lighter and easier to digest. Although those with Pitta constitutions can drink milk cold, both Kapha and Vata appreciate the warmth.

Additions to warm milk include ghee, sugar, honey, tea, or certain sweet or pungent spices. People with high cholesterol or those watching their weight can substitute skim milk and might avoid adding ghee to their warm milk.

## Milk Combinations

Milk—whether whole, skim, half and half, or heavy cream—is so full of nutritious qualities it is considered a whole food that digests best by itself. Except for such sweet and pungent foods as wheat, rice, sweet fruits, ginger, cayenne, and sweet- or pungent-tasting herbs that combine well with milk, AyurVeda, recommends that you enjoy milk by itself. Milk is not a good beverage to accompany dinner. Sugar, honey, wheat products, and other sweet-tasting ingredients aid in the digestion of milk. It is especially good to avoid mixing salty and sour foods with milk. Seafood and milk do not digest properly together.

## Some Milk-Based Beverages

These are a few milk-based beverages you might like to try at different times of the day. Enjoy them for breakfast, before bed, or as an afternoon snack, rather than with a meal. Although a somewhat cold and heavy for Kapha and Vata dieters, Fruit Smoothies are especially popular with those following a Pitta-reducing diet in summer. A tumbler of Fruit Smoothy made with a mixture of sweet fruits and a slice of buttered toast might make a satisfying light evening meal for Pitta when it's too hot to cook.

For an exceptionally satisfying and almost instantly Pitta-pacifying drink try Rose Petal Milkshake made from Maharishi Rose Petal Conserve. Vata and Kapha can drink it warm in any season.

## Rose Petal Milkshake

This elegant drink soothes and cools the fires of Pitta in summer. When served warm everyone can drink it year round. Rose petals are said to nourish the heart. When finished sipping the drink use a spoon to eat the remaining petals.

Makes 2 cups

> 2 cups milk—low fat for Kapha
> 1 1/2 tablespoons Rose Petal Conserve
> 1/4 teaspoon vanilla (optional)

Blend or shake thoroughly for 1 minute. The pieces of rose petals will settle to the bottom of the container. Take care to pour them all out when serving.

## Bed and Breakfast Drink

Good to drink in the morning and at bedtime.

> 1 cup milk per person— low fat for Kapha
> 1 to 2 teaspoons ghee
> Sugar to taste

Heat milk over moderate flame, stirring frequently. When just at boiling point add ghee and sugar. Stir and allow to come to a full boil. Cool and serve warm. For those reducing weight, eliminate the ghee and use skim milk.

## Saffron Milk Tea

This warm and rich drink is excellent for Vata. And, with modifications, it's good for Kapha, too. The saffron is a fine internal "heater," but it increases Pitta. In winter Pitta might enjoy a small amount of this drink.

For each serving:

> 1 cup milk
> 1 teaspoon ghee
> 1/2 teaspoon saffron, crumbled
> 1 teaspoon sugar

Heat milk in a heavy saucepan just to the boiling point. Add remaining ingredients and simmer for about 5 minutes or until the milk is rich yellow color. Cool and serve.

**For Kapha and Weight Watchers:** Use skim milk, omit the ghee, and reduce the sugar to taste.

## Indian Spiced Milk Tea

This tea is a fine afternoon pick-me-up and good for anyone who likes to drink black tea.

> 1 cup milk per serving
> 1 bag black tea per serving
> 1 to 2 teaspoons sugar
> 1/8 teaspoon ground cardamom
> 1/8 teaspoon cinnamon

Heat milk over moderate heat. When steamy add the other ingredients and stir frequently. Bring just to a boil. Cool before drinking.

**Note for Kapha:** Use skim or low fat milk and substitute ginger for the cardamom.

112

## Sweet Fruit Smoothies

This is a nourishing, cooling drink for balancing Pitta in the heat of summer. It is sweet, heavy, and cold when made with very ripe sweet fruits.

Mixing such different fruits as strawberries, peaches, bananas, kiwis, cherries, blueberries adds interest and flavor.

For each two-cup serving:

> 1 cup milk
> 1/2 cup ice cream (optional)
> 1 cup sliced ripe fruit
> 1 to 2 teaspoons sugar
> 1/4 teaspoon nutmeg or cinnamon (optional)
> 1/2 teaspoon vanilla

Whirl all ingredients in a blender or food processor or whisk by hand until blended.

## Three-in-One Samhita Supreme

The combination of spices, ghee, and milk in this drink make it so nourishing that it might be considered a rasayana. Good when served by itself for breakfast and again before bedtime. The first version is good for Vata and Pitta, the second is better for Kapha.

### I For Vata and Pitta

For each serving:

> 1 cup warm milk
> 1 teaspoon ghee
> 1 teaspoon sugar, or to taste
> 1/2 teaspoon of spices in this proportion:
> > 3 parts cardamom
> > 1 part cloves
> > 1 part cinnamon

Heat milk and ghee together and bring just to a boil. Stir in sugar and spices. Remove from heat and continue stirring until cool enough to drink. Make up a small batch of spices ahead of time and use 1/2 teaspoon spice mixture per cup of warm milk.

continues

## Three-in-One Samhita Supreme, continued

### II For Kapha

For each serving:

> 1 cup warm milk, skim milk best
> 1 teaspoon honey, or to taste
> 1 teaspoon of spices in this proportion:
>> 1 part cardamom
>> 1 part ground ginger
>> 1 part ground cloves
>> 1 part cinnamon

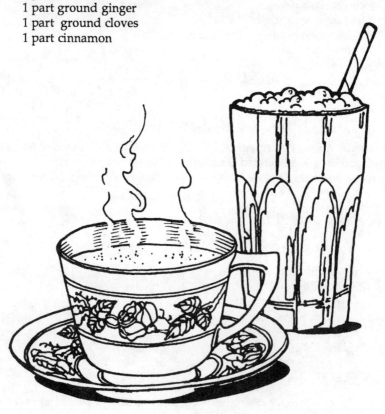

## Buttermilk and Lassi

Drinking buttermilk has gone out of style in America. It once was a healthful, popular beverage when we were a more rural country. But food interests seem to come and go, so perhaps the liking for buttermilk will return. Some people have never tasted it, or developed a taste for it. The commercial buttermilk that you buy from your local grocery store is fine to drink. Both Lassi (LAH-see), unflavored yogurt thinned with water to a drinking consistency, and buttermilk benefit all three constitutions in the same way. They make especially refreshing warm weather drinks.

> *I have never met anyone*
> *who could not drink Lassi.*
>
> - Dr. B. D. Triguna

These sour, cold, and heavy beverages decrease Vata but increase Pitta and Kapha, if taken in excess. They are best served alone as a fine thirst quenchers on a hot day, or at the end of a meal rather than in the beginning. Lassi should not be sipped along with a meal as if it were water. Taken alone, it is a nourishing food. Cold buttermilk, Lassi, or even large amounts of yogurt are not as healthful in cold weather as in warm. This is especially true for Vata and Kapha types. A small amount of salt, sugar, or such spices as ground cumin or ginger add to the taste.

## Plain Refreshing Lassi

Buttermilk, enhancing digestion in the same way as Lassi, can be substituted for yogurt and diluted with water to any consistency you like.

Makes 4 servings

    1 cup plain yogurt
    3 cups water

Place in cover container and shake vigorously.

## Cheese

Cottage cheese and most of the other kinds of cheese are good for Vata. Semisoft and hard cheese is too sour and aggravating for Pitta and Kapha digestions. Large quantities of hard cheese are difficult for all three types to digest. But such fresh, soft cheese as ricotta or panir can be eaten by everyone, even in moderation by Kapha types.

## Soft Cheese: Ricotta and Panir

Essentially, ricotta and panir are the same cheese except the first one comes from Italy and the other from India. Panir is usually the firmer of the two. It is possible to buy ricotta at many general grocery and specialty food stores. Good ricotta is made without stabilizers, gelatin, and additives. Read the label. Or, better yet, make your own.

## Curds

Making soft cheese is simply making curds and whey just as Little Miss Muffet may have done. The curds are the cheese part.

Makes 1 1/2 cups

> 2 quarts of milk
> 2 tablespoons lemon juice or white vinegar
> 1/2 cup yogurt (optional)

In a heavy pot bring milk to boil over moderately high heat. Watch it carefully so it doesn't boil over. As foam begins rising remove from heat and stir in juice or vinegar—and the yogurt, if it is used. Continue stirring gently as curds separate from whey. Set aside for 5 minutes and line a large sieve or colander with a loosely woven, clean towel or enough cheesecloth to tie into a bag.

Pour the cheese into the lined sieve, reserving the whey separately in lidded jars. Drain until cool. Then wrap the cloth tightly around the curds and squeeze out excess liquid. Hang the bag over a bowl or above the sink for an hour until most of the liquid is gone. Then press the cheese, slightly kneading it for panir, into a shallow pan or sealable container. Cover and refrigerate for 5 or 6 hours or overnight. Ricotta usually contains more liquid and is hung for less time, if at all. It does not have be kneaded and refrigerated, but can be used right away.

## And Whey

If you can take the time to make soft cheese you'll get the added benefit of whey, the clear, highly digestable liquid resulting from the cheese-making process. For a rich, nutty flavor, and added nutrition, substitute whey for the water in preparing rice and other grains. Or use it as a soup base, for some of the liquid in baking breads and cookies, or add some fresh chopped mint or other herbs or dosha balancing spices to warm whey and serve as a nutritious beverage. Try finding new uses for whey because it is too good to discard. Whey no longer has the protein and sweet properties of whole milk, so salt can be used in cooking with it.

## Honey, Molasses, and Sugar

Molasses, brown and white sugar including succanat, and honey are all fine for everyone to use to some extent. Sweeteners should be limited in diets for the overweight. Both molasses and honey contains heating properties so large amounts increase Pitta dosha. For that reason it is the sweetener of choice for Kapha. It tastes good mixed in warm or cool milk and herbal teas. Honey seems to carry the different herbal properties of the flowers it was gathered from and for that reason may have subtly differing effects depending on its origin.

*When the intensely sweet taste*
*of pure honey is on the tongue,*
*the taste of other sweets makes no impression.*

\- Maharishi Mahesh Yogi

Unlike sugar, honey has a couple of cautions to be followed when cooking. Honey should *never be heated* either by cooking, baking, or by adding it to boiling liquids. It can be safely added to liquids that have been heated then cooled to a warm temperature. If, over time, stored honey has become crystallized in the jar, warming it to pouring consistency in a pan of hot water from the tap is fine. Just don't boil it. Honey should not be mixed with equal amounts of ghee. This can result in skin problems.

## Whole Grains

Except for a few notations about quantities for each body type, everyone can include the following grains in a well-balanced diet unless they've been advised otherwise.

## Rice

Rice, an easily digested food for everyone's physical development, is sweet-tasting with cold, heavy qualities. It is such a versatile ingredient it should be a staple item in any kitchen. Two of the nicest things about cooking with rice are that it absorbs the flavors of liquids and spices prepared with it and complements almost any main dish in a meal.

## Basmati: the Queen of All Rice

For the AyurVedic rice should unfailingly result in attractively separate grains, never be sticky, display the longest grain possible, and have a delicious, uniquely nutty flavor. The only rice that matches this description is Basmati, the standard by which all other rices are measured, the queen of all rice.

According to Dr. Bill D. Webb, of the United States Department of Agriculture and foremost rice expert in the U.S., there are two types of Basmati, authentic Punjabi Basmati and all its imitators. In its raw state premium Basmati appears as a very fine, polished, slender grain. But the unusual thing about this rice is that when cooked it elongates more than 200% of its original size. Basmati has the natural capacity to absorb more water than other long-grain rice. This ability to absorb water keeps it from becoming sticky. And it always has a distinctive flavor.

For some time the USDA has tried to grow Basmati rice but they have not been able to reproduce the same unique flavor or the elongating properties. Dr. Webb thinks it might be because of the specific laws of nature in its growing environment, the Punjab of India, have yet to be found in the U.S. or elsewhere in the world.

## Other Rices

Other long-grain rices might be called Basmati II. One of these is called Texmati. Widely available in natural food stores, it is a cross between Basmati and American long-grain rice. Although sometimes sold as Basmati, it is considered simply as a good long-grain rice. There are also California and Thailand "Basmati" types available, but they do not have the authentic flavor and length when cooked. These are all nutritious and less expensive substitutes, however. Reconstituted and "processed" instant type rices are not.

Sweet rice is a very short grain rice that can be found in oriental grocery stores. It makes an unforgettably rich pudding. Wild rice is a tasty, dark, long grain that is not stirctly speaking a true rice, but more of a nutty-flavored substitute. It is not as easy to digest as other rice. Brown rice, or red rice as it is known in AyurVeda, is a healthful rice good for body building and general nutrition. Although not always considered as tasty as polished Basmati, with its outer layer of bran intact it is richer in fiber and vitamins. In some countries brown rice and other of the more nutritious whole grains are fed to cows more often than to people.

## Rice for Kapha and Weight Reducing

Everyone can benefit from eating rice, but people with Kapha constitutions should fry the washed rice grains in a little ghee or oil until they are transparent, then the rice can be cooked as usual. This gives the rice a lighter quality that Kapha types appreciate. People watching their weight should eat less rice because it builds all tissues, including fat.

## Wheat

Wheat, another sweet food that is good for all aspects of nutrition, can be eaten by everyone except people inclined to have colitis. Wheat does not cause allergies. Something growing with the wheat may cause reactions in some people. If someone thinks he has a wheat allergy or an allergy related to any of the foods mentioned here he should consult an AyurVedic physician.[3]

Wheat comes in a wide variety of flours, shapes, and forms. Whole wheat and unbleached white flours are the most nutritious for everyday baking. Semolina wheat makes wonderful pastas and couscous. Dry breakfast cereals of wheat—sometimes mixed with rice and oats—make good morning or evening light meals and digestible foods while fasting. Not as widely used, bulgar, a traditional Middle Eastern grain of cracked wheat berries, is available at natural food stores and many supermarkets. Kasha, the roasted kernels, or groats, is treated as a grain but is actually the fruit of the buckwheat plant. It is high in digestible protein and very good for building muscles, tissue, and, in excess, fat, for Vata and Pitta. The process of toasting kasha lightens it, making it good for Kapha in moderation.

## Barley

Even though barley, whether used as a flour, or boiled unhulled or pearled, is not as nutritious as other grains, it has a light quality that is easily digested. Barley is so good for Kapha body types that it should be their "grain of choice" and eaten frequently. Barley has very little fat or sodium, making it an

119

especially good rice substitute for those needing to lose weight. When served as a main dish or the major part of the meal, barley is too light in quality to satisfy the needs of Pitta and Vata, as rice and wheat do. Some cooks find it is more versatile than wheat or rice. For all body types, barley is useful in preventing constipation. The water left from cooking whole barley has diuretic properties. It can also be used as a base in making vegetable soups.

Stuffed green peppers with herbed barley or a simple sauté of barley tossed with some favorite steamed vegetables are satisfying foods for weight watchers. Without changing the result, barley flour can replace up to one third of the wheat flour in a bread recipe, making it more edible for Kapha types. It is a good basic grain to prepare for those recovering from illness. AyurVeda considers barley a food for the prevention of illness when included as part of a well-balanced diet.

## Corn and Millet

Whole corn, and cornmeal used in baking, are nourishing for everyone, especially for those with Kapha constitutions. Its heating properties make it less appetizing for Pitta, especially in summer. Cornbread, or cornmeal mixed with other grains in bread, helps to reduce fat.

Millet is a sweet whole grain, a staple of African cookery, but served most frequently in America as birdseed. It's versatile enough to substitute for other grains when we want to add more variety to meals. Millet also makes an easily digested, warm breakfast cereal healthy for everyone.

## Lentils

Lentils, also called pulses or gram, are available either polished and split or whole. They can be made into a soup with vegetables and herbs, or cooked alone into a thick broth known as dahl (sounds like "doll"). To make a nutritionally balanced entree dahl is usually served with rice . In a vegetarian diet lentils provide an easy way to maintain a proper balance of protein and essential mineral and trace elements. Adding an astringent taste to a meal, they are especially recommended for Pitta and Kapha diets. The lentils listed in this book can be found in most natural food or Asian grocery stores. There are interesting and subtle differences in the flavors of each type, and it can be fun to experiment with them. Whole lentils require soaking for a couple of hours before cooking. If you are in a hurry, split lentils cook much faster than the whole gram. Yellow or green split peas are available at most grocery stores. They can be substituted in the recipes calling for lentils, but the consistency and flavor of pea soup remain identifiable.

## Quick and Delicious Dahl

Another speedy and altogether healthy AyurVedic cooking suggestion is to prepare lentils, as well as rice or vegetables, in a pressure cooker. Lentils can be cooked into a soup prior to preparing the vegetables or other parts of the meal, and then heated again just before serving. Reheat leftover lentil and bean dishes by frying in hot oil. A little salt and seasonings can turn a rather bland pot of boiled lentils into a tasty soup or dahl.

One of the easiest seasonings to use in making an authentic Indian dahl is Maharishi Vata Churna. It is a special blend of spices most healthful for Vata types and everyone else in cold, windy weather.

Another way to cook unsplit lentils is by frying. Sprouted lentils, that is, whole gram soaked in tepid water until just ready to sprout, are delicious when fried in oil or ghee. All lentils, beans, and unprocessed rice should be picked over carefully to remove any little stones, and then washed very well, usually in three changes of cool water.

There are many popular whole and split lentils to choose from for making dahl. Most are available at Asian groceries or natural food stores.

## Green Mung Gram

These are the same little beans sprouted for use in Chinese cooking. When served as a very liquid soup, whole mung bean dahl is good for everyone. If a person has excellent digestion, that is, very active agni, a mung dahl of a more solid, thick consistency can be eaten. Prepared in this way it is a good food for ending a long fast, or when feeling particularly ravenous.

## Split Mung

Split mung lentils cook more quickly than the whole bean and do not cause gas when thoroughly cooked. When properly prepared, in its most most digestible state, Mung Dahl should look very creamy.

## Chana Lentils

Also called split chick peas, Chana lentils are light, rich tasting, and easy to digest. This dahl is also a good food to eat in cases of diarrhea.

121

## Toor Dahl

When bought at an Indian grocery store these split pigeon peas appear a shiny, golden yellow. They are covered in oil for preservation. Before cooking, the oil must be thoroughly washed off under very hot water. Richly delicious, Toor dahl can be a regular part of everyone's diet.

## Urad Gram

Whole Urad (OOR-ad) beans are sold as black lentils that look like very small black beans. They should not be confused with black turtle beans, which even though small are about twice as large as Urad beans. The inside of the bean is pure white and rather oily. Cooking Urad dahl takes about twice as long as any other; but they make a rich, hearty, exceptionally nutritious soup. Sprouted and fried is the best way for Kapha types to eat whole Urad. An excellent body building food for Vata and Pitta, Urad gram can be eaten by those needing to put on weight and muscles, and, it is said, for ladies wishing to have "excellent offspring."

## Urad Lentils

These are the black urad beans that have been skinned and split in half. They are very good for everyone, especially for those with Vata and Pitta constitutions. White lentils act as a tonic and general body builder. Eating too much Urad dahl, however, increases Kapha. These lentils cook faster than the whole Urad beans, are just as nutritious, and benefit from the addition of turmeric for a richer color.

## Masoor Lentils

The fastest cooking of all lentils, bright coral-colored masoor also has somewhat less nutritional value than the others. But they only take about 15 minutes to make.

## Muth Lentils

These are the flat, brown-colored lentils commonly found in supermarkets. They can be cooked into a stew or dahl as other lentils, or prepared as a hearty and unusual breakfast food, or a side dish at a regular meal, by frying just-sprouted muth lentils in a little oil or ghee with a choice of "dosha-appropriate" spices, then served with rice.

## Dried Beans

AyurVeda gives a general guideline for eating dishes cooked with dried beans. Once a week is enough for anyone. Beans are body building and hard to digest at the same time. Most beans are all right for Kapha and Pitta, but they do aggravate Vata. Although Pitta is increased somewhat by eating beans, the increase is not significant, except, of course, for spicy chili beans. Because of their heavy body-building nature, eating too many bean dishes increases Kapha. Soybeans and soybean products, including tofu, are fine for Vata and Pitta types, but because of their cold, heavy, sometimes oily qualities, they increase Kapha. For Vata constitutions eating beans once a week is enough. For Kapha, eating a dish containing tofu once a week is plenty. During Kapha season tofu can be eliminated from the menu for those subject to colds or bronchial problems, and general feelings of sluggishness.

## Fruits

The best fresh fruits for daily consumption are apples, sweet oranges, melons (in season)—especially that summertime favorite, watermelon. Dried dates, raisins, and figs are good for everyone. AyurVeda says they bring a feeling of fulfillment and satisfaction. Even though "dried" they are neither dry in quality nor too drying for Vata and Pitta to enjoy fully, but the sweet taste is concentrated in dried fruits so eating too many will increase Kapha.

## Ghee and Other Oils

Ghee is refined clarified butter. Both a rasayana and an auspicious food of the superior category, ghee is the first choice in cooking oils. It can be made from any kind of butter but that from cow's milk is the best. For medicinal purposes, AyurVeda uses a specially refined ghee that has been heated and filtered many times. Simply refined ghee, well-filtered once, is used for cooking. When properly made ghee needs no refrigeration, since there are no milk solids left in it to spoil. Unopened ghee has a shelf life of two years.

*Ghee maintains youth.*
*Some ghee every day prevents aging.*
- Dr. T. M. Gopte

## To Make Cooking Ghee

In a heavy saucepan melt a pound or more of butter over medium heat. When butter becomes liquid and foamy turn the heat to low. Simmer slowly for about an hour, skimming the froth off every once in a while. Unless the ghee is made from fresh, unsalted butter (not the commercial variety) discard the skimmings. Otherwise these are a nutritious addition to rice, bread, or dahl.

When the ghee turns a golden yellow and little brown bits of milk solids lie at the bottom of the pan, it is ready to be filtered into a clean jar.

Pour it through a fine sieve lined with a coffee filter. Lacking a paper filter, the fine sieve will do. A double sieve is even better. It is not necessary to refrigerate ghee when all the milk solids have been removed, but keep it tightly covered after using.

## Ghee and Cholesterol

Ghee and vegetable oils, when properly used, do not increase cholesterol. Long term AyurVedic research in India indicates that the regular use of ghee in the diet presupposes a normally active life, and when it is used in combination with certain sweet or pungent spices ghee and other vegetable oils help balance the diet and maintain good agni. The researchers say that adding these spices enables the body to use the oils more efficiently and avoid high cholesterol levels. The best spices to heat in ghee are ground cumin, hing (asafoetida), ground coriander seeds, tumeric, and ground fenugreek. These

124

should be heated in the oil, then added to the rest of a recipe. If you have questions about diet and cholesterol consult your physician.

## Chocolate

Even though chocolate can be enjoyed in moderation, it is not one of those ingredients recommended wholeheartedly for everyone. This seems to be as good a place as any to say a few words about one of our favorite—some would claim essential—American treats.

There is concern among health enthusiasts that the alkali used when processing chocolate into baking cocoa as well as the liqueur for candy making renders the product alkaline. Eating alkaline foods vitiates or weakens all doshas. Alkali is used in processing highly refined European cocoa ( called the Dutch process), thought by gourmets to be the best quality cocoa available. The good news is that quality baking chocolate, not processed with alkali, is available at your supermarket. It's good old American Hershey's chocolate.

Of course you may purchase your own cocoa beans[4], roast, and grind them yourself. You'll obtain a crumbly, slightly gritty cocoa outstanding in making hot chocolate and general baked goods. For those concerned about alkaline in the diet, the amount of alkaline in a slice of cake made with imported chocolate is significantly less than that found in a glass of carbonated soda.

AyurVeda's greater interest in chocolate has to do with the quantity consumed weekly, daily, (hourly?) in the contemporary American diet. Chocolate is a bitter, astringent-tasting ingredient that increases Vata, and if eaten in moderation decreases Pitta and Kapha. Sweetened chocolate increases Kapha. This does not mean chocolate is to be eliminated from the diet, only that everyone who cares to eat chocolate should do so moderately, in this case, once every week or two is frequent enough, not daily.

AyurVeda does not consider carob as a substitute for chocolate. Certain properties in carob beans are thought to contribute to illness.

## Spices For Everyone

The Maharishi Ayur-Veda Churnas are special blends of herbs and spices that promote health as well as add flavor to your cooking. They can be used as garam masala when following Indian recipes. Most of time that means they can be heated in a little oil or ghee then added to cooked vegetables to make a "curried" dish. Or they can be mixed in small amounts with any of your favorite foods to taste. All three churnas—Vata, Pitta, and Kapha can be used by everyone to some extent. This, too, depends on taste and individual seasonal needs. In addition to enhancing dahls each of the churnas provides rich and marvelous flavorings for creamy soups, gravies, marinades, dressings, and sauces. Experiments with these churnas yield many pleasant results. They can be ordered directly from Maharishi AyurVeda Products International listed in back of the book.

## Best Use of the Churnas

The Maharishi Churnas come in handy when you want to be certain all six tastes—sweet, salty, sour, bitter, astringent, and pungent—are represented in a meal. When a main meal is AyurVedically balanced, meaning that each of the six tastes can be clearly identified, then the entire meal is balanced. So, the Churnas should not be sprinkled over an entire plate of food. Nor should a single Churna be used in every dish. This blurs or throws off the effect of the different tastes and the balance in the meal. Add a single Churna to only one or two dishes at a meal. Then use a different one, other herbs or spices, or just the combined ingredients themselves to make good-tasting, well-balanced meals.

Although the following spices may increase certain doshas, they are still considered good for everyone when used moderately in the regular diet.

## Asafoetida (Hing)

A powerful smelling, resin-like spice, hing is both astringent and heating in the stomach after eating. It is a good intestinal antiseptic and, therefore, very good for Vata. Hing should not be used by itself but fried with other spices in a little oil and then put in dahl (the best way to use it) or with mixed vegetables. For use in dahl, put a pinch of hing in the boiling water just before adding the lentils and cover quickly to keep the strong essence in the steam and not all over the kitchen. Lentil and bean dishes should always be made with a pinch of hing to aid digestion. Too much hing aggravates Pitta. When using Vata Churna to flavor dahl it is not necessary to add hing, it is in the Churna.

## Coriander

Freshly ground seeds are best when fried in hot oil and added to vegetable dishes, rice, or soups. They are sweet, slightly pungent, and oily. The leaves of the coriander plant, cilantro, add pungent, astringent, and bitter tastes to salads and vegetable dishes. Cilantro is also good for everyone.

## Cumin

To get the best taste from cumin seeds, dry roast them in a small pan, then grind into a powder. With sweet, bitter, pungent, and light aspects, cumin compliments tomato-based dishes. It is a basic spice for Vata diet.

## Nutmeg

Nutmeg goes nicely with dairy products, cooked fruits, vegetables, and dahls. AyurVeda recommends increasing the use of nutmeg in the diet during hay fever season. When added to warm milk nutmeg promotes sleep (as does the milk). Rice made with ghee and nutmeg has superior eating qualities.

## Turmeric

A brilliant yellow powder, turmeric is always heated in oil before mixing with other ingredients. A unifying herb, when cooked with other spices turmeric tends to pull all the flavors of a dish together. AyurVeda thinks of turmeric as a good blood purifier and skin tonic. It is slightly bitter, astringent, and pungent.

## Cardamom

Sweet, bitter, and astringent ground cardamom is at its best when heated with milk, included in sweet main dishes, and in baking sweet breads and cookies. Kapha types should use less than others. It makes a good spice for a warming winter drink.

## The Best of the Best

Certain foods are so especially nutritious that AyurVeda has identified them as "rasayanas"—foods that promote longevity. A rasayana (rah-SY-uh-nah) contains all the nutrition needed for the development of every body tissue. It works on that familiar gardening principle of watering the root of a plant to develop all the parts. Rasayanas nourish the very basis of physical life.

A plump, light-colored fig known as *anjier* is a rasayana for everyone. It is sold in some supermarkets and natural food stores as a white Calmyrna fig. In AyurVeda *anjier* is called "the rasayana of all fruit." Other rasayanas include Basmati rice, ghee, wheat, Urad beans, blanched almonds, and nutmeg.

## Notes:

[1]All the recipes and food recommendations in this book are for the general population. People with diabetes or other medically restricted diets should follow their doctor's advice.

[2] To order Maharishi Ayur-Veda Products call 1-800-ALL-VEDA.

[3]See listing of Maharishi Ayur-Veda Physicians of North America.

[4]Fresh Mexican cocoa beans available by the pound with preparation instructions from J. L. Hudson, Seedsman, P. O. Box 1058. Redwood City, CA  94064.

Chapter 7

# In the AyurVedic Kitchen

## An AyurVedic Kitchen

An "Ayurvedic" kitchen is simply a clean, well-equipped food preparation area located away from the center of household traffic. It is a quiet place where the colors of the walls and cabinets, comfortable flooring, the room size and ease of getting around, and even the view out of a window all contribute to the cook's general sense of well-being. This, in turn, is subtly reflected in the kind of food prepared there.

Like any creative workspace an AyurVedic kitchen should be simple, well-lighted and ventilated, orderly, and easy to keep clean. When stepping into the AyurVedic cook's kitchen the atmosphere should feel calm, pleasant, and pure . . . and be filled with deliciously enticing smells. Outdoor clothing and shoes are not worn there. Whenever possible, only the cook and those involved in food preparation should be in the kitchen while cooking.

## First, Prepare the Cook

Preparation of a good AyurVedic meal involves more than producing something to eat. Of course the cook collects all the ingredients, washes, chops, stirs, fries, bakes, and so forth to make something that becomes more than just the collection of assorted ingredients. With every thoughtful meal as an AyurVedic cook you are preparing a special gift, a *yagya* ,for those who are to eat. But the AyurVedic meal really begins ahead of time and, most importantly, with the preparation of the cook.

*Food is affected
by the tendencies of the cook
who prepares it.*

- Maharishi Mahesh Yogi

A fully prepared cook is satisfied in mind and body. Meditate, even briefly, and then eat something just before you begin cooking a large meal. Transcendental Meditation is part of modern day AyurVeda. By regularly practicing the TM program the cook naturally feels calm and orderly while working. Even though there may be many dishes to prepare or lots of steps to follow in a recipe, a sense of restful alertness while working allows you to be more consciously aware of all that goes into a successful meal.

And by eating something like tea and toast, a sandwich, or piece of fruit before beginning to cook, you can avoid tasting the food excessively and be less tempted to save some out for yourself before serving it. Such rather greedy thoughts affect the food, causing dissatisfaction in those who eat it. This is because the quality of the cook's consciousness is carried by the food itself.

*Food prepared by a loving*
*settled, sattvic cook*
*creates loving, settled, sattvic people.*

\- Nancy Lonsdorf, M.D.

## The Cook's Attention

The cook's thoughts and feelings affect all parts of the meal. For this reason one should neither cook nor eat when angry or upset. The quality of the cook's attention has as much to do with the success of a meal as all of the ingredients and any utensils you use. To maintain your attention avoid such distractions as listening to music, having long telephone conversations, playing the radio or television, chatting with visitors, or anything that keeps you from thinking about the job at hand.

When cooking like this you become more aware of the various parts of meal preparation, including appetizing color combinations, the proper balance of taste and qualities for each dish, as well as the needs of each the people who will be eating. When you enjoy such an intensely creative cooking process in this way anything else will seem like an unwelcome distraction.

In the quiet of the kitchen you naturally consider everything that is to be used—all the fruits and vegetables, spices, oils, and grains, and how they all are to be handled to achieve the desired results. And your attention goes beyond the kitchen as you think affectionately of those who will be eating what you prepare.

## Fresh is Best

AyurVeda says, "Fresh is always best." Foods are delivered to us from all parts of the country, usually over long distances. Although it would be wonderful, not all "fresh" foods are garden fresh or even locally grown. But finding and using the freshest ingredients, grown without pesticides and properly stored, should be an AyurVedic cook's goal. The cook's real responsibility for the quality of the ingredients begins when they are brought into the kitchen. It's worthwhile to begin a little garden near your kitchen and grow the herbs and vegetables you like most to eat.

*When you grow an AyurVedic kitchen garden*
*you enjoy the best fresh produce*
*right at your doorstep.*

## Leftovers

Fresh ingredients freshly prepared are better for everyone than old leftovers. When the main meal is eaten at noon or a little after, as is best, certain leftovers can be stored in the refrigerator or a cool place and reheated in the evening, or, at the very latest, for breakfast. This includes rice and whole grain dishes not containing vegetables or dairy products, lentil dahls, lassi, undressed salads, and fruits cooked with sugar. After that there are simply not enough active ingredients in the food to make eating it worthwhile.

When preparing beans, grains, and dahls left from the previous meal, heat them very well by frying in oil or ghee rather than boiling again. Cooked vegetables and unsweetened cooked fruits do not keep well as leftovers.

## Cook Plentifully

Even if you cook simply always cook plentifully as you can. There should be more than enough food prepared for everyone. Sitting down to eat with feelings of abundance and a welcome invitation to enjoy it all makes for happiness and satisfaction in everyone at the table. This is not a recommendation for extravagance or waste, however. In the AyurVedic view, food is a blessing not to be wasted. Extra cooked food should be given to a neighbor or friend in need, or as a special treat to someone who you think would enjoy it. As a gift of bounty, always send enough food not only for your friend, but an extra amount so he can have a guest.

*Food should not be wasted.*
*Always cook more than enough.*
*And, if there are leftovers, send them to*
*someone who needs them.*
*Send enough for the needy person and his guest.*

- Dr. P. D. Subhedar

## Cleanliness

Meal preparation includes cleaning, cutting and chopping, mixing and heating, and food storage. It is important to keep the work area clean. Washing the hands before beginning, after handling soiled things, and frequently while cooking are healthy habits. It is also important to regularly wash all parts of the kitchen surfaces well with a mild bleach solution of about one teaspoon bleach per gallon of water. This is especially useful in preventing bacterial build-up on wooden cutting boards and spoons. The solution is so mild it does not affect food tastes.

In addition to washing fruits and vegetables before using them, whole spices, lentils, and grains, including non-enriched or imported rice, should also be sorted and cleansed. They can often hide little stones or twigs. Wash rice, beans, and grains in cool water, rinsing two or three times, or until the water runs clear.

*Good cooking is not a matter of fast or slow time.*
*Just cook the food for as long*
*as needed until it's done.*
*No more no less.*

- Dr. H. S. Kasture

## Heating

Cooking is a lot like performing chemistry experiments. The ingredients have chemical components. Heating them can change the food properties and cause chemical interactions that sometimes alter the effect of the original raw ingredients. By heating water, milk, and some other foods, heavy elements are made lighter and easier to digest. Cold foods are heavy and congestive to the stomach, slowing digestion. By cooking such foods as cabbage and apples they become easier for the stomach to convert into useful active ingredients than when they are served raw either by themselves or in salad. Certain foods should not be cooked together, such as fish and milk, or milk with either lemon juice or salt. These combinations generally cause imbalances, as do equal amounts of ghee and honey mixed together.

## Cooking Methods

Of the most commonly used heating methods steaming, boiling, frying, grilling, and baking are best. Of these, steam is the very best way to preserve the most nutrients, especially those in vegetables, fruits, and whole grains. AyurVeda does not recommend microwave cookery because it is thought that the process rearranges the active food ingredients, making their effects unpredictable. Good efficient cooking is not necessarily a matter of speed. But neither is AyurVedic cooking a tedious, slow process with the cook spending a long time stirring the pot and thinking about putting her best attention into the food. The AyurVedic cook just heats things for as long as they need to be cooked without making a mood of it by slowing the process down or rushing to get the meal done at the expense of the nourishing value of the food.

## Faster Cooking: A Pressure Cooker

If getting a meal cooked and served quickly is important, then try a pressure cooker. By using steam heat, pressure cooking is a fast, healthful way to cook a variety of foods simultaneously. An entire meal can be prepared in a few minutes in a pressure cooker. For a rice and mixed vegetable dinner simply layer rice on the bottom of the pan with a proper amount of water and add your choice of vegetables cut into pieces of equal size. Follow manufacturer's directions for length of time to cook rice The seasonings can be adjusted before serving. This is a cooking method that holds appeal for busy professionals and families who don't have time to fuss but want to serve highly nutritious meals. Cooking a mixed meal in a pressure cooker also has the advantage of allowing the cook to season the different foods as they are finished cooking according to each family member's needs.

## Food Storage

In an AyurVedic cook's kitchen the refrigerator is rarely filled to capacity. If you opened the freezer you might find ice cubes, ice cream, nuts, flours, grains, and extra spices in cold storage, but little else. Frozen foods, even milk, have altered molecular qualities and offer less or uncertain nutrition. Since we don't eat ice cream primarily for its nutritional value, freezing it hardly matters. But cooking up large batches of food and freezing them for later use is not nutritionally practical, even though it seems to save time. Either canned and frozen foods can be used as garnishes, or they may make up a small proportion of a dish. Eating frozen or canned meals might be all right once every week or two, but these foods should not make up the greater proportion of the diet.

*First, select fresh foods,*
*that are locally grown,*
*and in season.*

## Food Storage: How to Use a Refrigerator

Even the refrigerator in an AyurVedic cook's kitchen is mostly empty of fresh produce or leftovers. For the most part just chill whatever vegetables and fruits necesssary for the next meals, as well as those basic dairy products that keep for a few days. Refrigerators of today are cold, closed systems that allow the slow deterioration of food. They would be more useful for storage if they had air exchange systems. Without ventilation, as one food spoils everything else follows or is affected by the spoilage. However, refrigerators are good for long term storage of items that are kept in sealed containers such as nuts, nut butters, pickles and other condiments, salad dressings, jams, andfruit preserves.

It is important regularly, about every week or two, to empty the refrigerator of fresh produce and anything stored for long periods of time and wash the interior thoroughly with a mild bleach solution.

## Storing Root Crops

The best way to store such root crops as potatoes, parsnips, and sweet potatoes is in a cool, dark, ventilated cabinet. Replacing the doors on a kitchen cabinet with a decorative lattice or screen would allow enough ventilation if it is located in a cool place.

## Storing Flours and Other Grains

An exception to the concept of food storage for freshness is the AyurVedic guideline for storing wheat and rice. "Old" wheat and rice, that is, rice and wheat that have been carefully stored for two to four years, have more nutrition available in them than new wheat or rice. But freshly ground flour is preferred and seems to hold the most flavor. As a rule, use any ground flour within two months after purchase or milling. After that it deteriorates quickly. Just before using flour, sift it or stir it well to air it.

Store flour, other grains, nuts, and other foods in tightly covered plastic, ceramic, glass, or stainless steel containers. The only disadvantage to glass for food storage is that it chips and breaks easily. To be sure of freshness you might want to refrigerate or freeze flours and grains.

## Equipment and Utensils

The best kitchen utensils and equipment are those tools the cook feels most comfortable using. Use cooking equipment that does not reduce or alter the active nutritional ingredients in the food. It is best to avoid cooking and storing food in metals that cause chemical reactions, such as aluminium, plastic-or teflon-coated, or chipped enamel. Copper pans should be used only for boiling drinking water. Copper-clad pan bottoms conduct heat very well and are good on stainless steel pans, but copper should never come into contact with food. Recommended materials for casserole dishes, pots, and pans are stainless steel, well-seasoned carbon steel, cast iron, and glass. Either stainless steel or wooden spoons and utensils are best choices. Use a separate spoon for each dish being prepared. since one spoon used for all the cooking transfers the flavors from one pot to another and muddles the individual tastes.

## Cooking for a Group

When judging the consistency of a dish, it should be the most easily digestible and balancing for the specific type of person who will be eating it. Thick soups, dahls, and even some milk-based drinks are not easy for Vata and Kapha types to digest. It is better to dilute them and adjust the seasonings accordingly. Most people with Pitta constitutions can easily digest thick foods, or just about anything else. If you are serving a group of people with varied dietary needs always prepare the more easily digestible versions of a recipe and provide a varied selection of tastes and qualites so there's something for everyone.

## The Moment of Judgement

There comes a point in the preparation of a meal when the cook needs to make a judgement about the overall tastes and consistencies of each dish. In tasting the food take a small amount out of the pan and taste it. It is not necessary or desirable to frequently taste the food during cooking. Taste only when it seems to be finished, or there is a question about its effect. With experience the tasting of the food before serving becomes a rare necessity.

## Adjusting Seasonings

Tasting for a balance of seasonings, or "adjusting" the seasonings, means sampling the most liquid part of the dish and making changes as necessary. Take a small spoonful and, as it passes over the tongue to the throat, notice which of the six tastes are most outstanding or where the sensation of taste occurs. If you've cooked something spicy the predominant sensation will be in the back of the throat. When a dish is rich in flavors the tastes will enliven many parts of the palate. One well-prepared entree can deliciously satisfy the six essential taste requirements for a balanced meal, and it will be a memorable experience for everyone eating it.

## Just Before Serving

The final judgement comes when the cook looks at the many finished dishes and takes a kind of mental inventory to see that all of the tastes, qualities, and categories are represented. At this point some last minute adjustments can be made by adding condiments, pickles, or perhaps a quickly prepared warm side dish to balance the meal further and increase the variety. Add a little more of the bitter taste with a bouquet of shortened celery sticks with the leaves left on, or some sour coolness with a bowl of lime and lemon wedges, or a small bowl of wilted lettuce (chopped lettuce, quickly sautéed in hot oil with minced ginger). It's handy for making up any pungent and slightly bitter tastes that may be missing. And then serve the dinner with pride and be ready to accept all the justified compliments you'll receive.

*Every kitchen should be filled*
*with appetizing smells.*
*Then when the guests arrive*
*they can't help but say,*
*"Everything smells great."*
*Without other appetizers*
*they are ready to eat.*

\- Dr. P. D. Subhedar

# 7  The AyurVeda Cookbook

*Chapter 8*

# *The AyurVeda Gourmet*

## Dining

An AyurVedic meal is a time for enjoyment and celebration. When food is eaten at the right time, in a pleasant setting, with good company, and in the proper quantity, then eating becomes one of the best experiences in life. AyurVeda offers a few simple guidelines for good eating.

## Atmosphere

Meals should be enjoyed in a clean, calm setting. Even the simplest dinner for two can be a celebration filled with laughter and good feelings, quiet music, or companionable silence. When dining alone silence or some agreeable dinner music is the best accompaniment for good digestion.

*Food is affected by the tendencies*
*of the mind and quality of thoughts*
*while it is being eaten.*
*So the frame of mind*
*in which one eats and the company and*
*conversation at the time*
*are highly important.*
-Maharishi Mahesh Yogi

## Conversation

Table conversation is light and entertaining for everyone. No unpleasant or weighty topics should be discussed. Mealtime is not the time to make decisions (exit the "business lunch"). Discuss business or other important matters after eating. Positive decisions can be made when everyone is feeling well satisfied by a good meal. Conversation includes listening to others and not talking and chewing food at the same time.

## Interruptions

Avoid visitors, telephone, television, loud music, reading, and other distractions while eating. The benefit of a good meal comes from eating with your full attention. Ask unexpected visitors to join you at your meal or make arrangements to meet with them after eating. Meals should not be eaten while driving a car or during other activities.

## Sit Comfortably

Sit down to eat. . .always. It is best for proper digestion to sit when eating. The stomach is in the best position for digestion when there is a little pressure on it. Standing while eating or drinking gives the wrong message to the stomach, and because there is not enough pressure the food flows through too fast. The one responsible for serving the food should have either already eaten, or else have all the food conveniently located so no one has to get up and down to help others during the meal.

At the end of a meal sit for 5 or 10 minutes and relax.

## Time

Eat when you are hungry, after the previous meal is completely digested. Take the time to eat well. The age-old advice of taking your time to chew your food well still applies. Just before eating pause for a moment or two and sit in silence with the eyes closed to allow the doshas to settle; or use that silent time for a brief prayer.

*Praise the food served to you, never criticize it.*
*Food is Brahman.*
*Food is the Self.*

-The Upanishads

## Best Time For Dinner: Midday

Invite guests to a special dinner at the midday meal rather than at night. According to AyurVeda the noon meal is the most substantial one of the day. Everyone's digestive juices function best when the sun is at its peak. In the evening and after sunset heavy food is not digested as well. Eat a light meal then.

## How To Eat: Layers Of Food And Water

Eat to two-thirds of your capacity. Sip small amounts of water while eating. One third of the meal should be water and one third solid food. The final third of the stomach is left empty to leave room for the action of digestion. Eat just until you feel satisfied, but not "full." Eating too much food gives pressure to the heart and can cause heartburn or gas.

## Signs Of A Good Ayurvedic Meal

Food is well-prepared with the cook's full attention.
It is presented promptly with appetizing colors.
It smells, feels, and tastes delicious.
The setting is comfortable, clean, pleasant.
Everyone eats with a good appetite.

### After the Meal

Feel increased mental energy,
comfort and strength,
clarity of senses.
Feeling of satisfaction and well-being.

Parties and Celebrations

Whether simple or elaborate
every AyurVedic meal is a party.
The menus in this section
have an international flavor that
for many of us means celebrating.
When entertaining people with varied
dietary needs serve these meals buffet style,
there's something here for everyone
to enjoy.

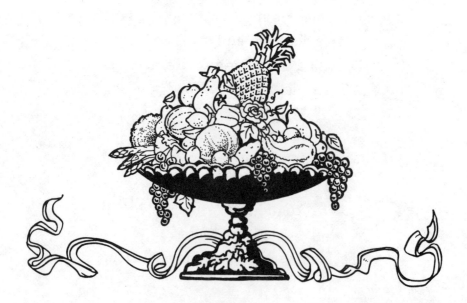

## An Indian Feast

A complete meal of Indian-style food is balanced by tastes and qualities. Everything is offered in abundance. It is for each person to choose the appropriate amount of each dish according to the season and individual preference. There are more recipes listed in this menu than you would usually cook at one meal. For an impressive feast the basic dahl, rice, bread, and vegetable dish can be enhanced by making many chutneys and condiments. An Indian feast begins with a tradtional blessing.

*Saha nav avatu*

*Saha nau bhunaktu*

*Saha viryam karavavhai*

*Tejasvi nav adhitam astu*

*Ma vidvishavahai*

-The Upanishads

Let us be together

Let us eat together

Let us be vital together

Let us be radiating truth,

Radiating the light of life,

Never shall we denounce anyone

Never entertain negativity

# AN INDIAN MENU

### MASOOR DAHL AND RICE
(Astringent, Sweet, Dry, Cold )

### SPICED VEGETABLE CURRY
(Pungent, Sour, Sweet, Slightly Bitter, Astringent, Salty, Hot)
or
### SWEET CURRY AND SAFFRON RICE
(Sweet, Salty, Astringent)

### RAITAS
(Sour, Cold, Salty )

### CHUTNEYS AND OTHER CONDIMENTS

### PURIS OR CHAPATIS
(Sweet, Heavy )

### CASHEW NUT BALLS
(Sweet, Oily, Slightly Heavy)

### FRAGRANT SPICED LASSI
(Sour, Sweet, Cold )

## Masoor Dahl

Dahl, a rich lentil soup, is best for all of your guests when it is made in a very liquid consistency. Eating dahl is good for people of all body types. For more information about other lentils used in making dahl see Chapter 6, "Something For Everyone." Masoor Dahl, made from thin, coral-colored lentils, cooks faster than any others.

Although dahl can be made with various spice combinations, an easy and most delicious way is by using the Maharishi Ayur-veda Product, Vata Churna. This combination of spices never fails to produce a rich and authentically Indian dahl.

Serves 4 to 6

    5 cups water
    1 cup red lentils
    1 tablespoon ghee
    1 teaspoon salt, or to taste
    1 tablespoon Vata Churna
            or
    Choice of ground spices and a pinch of hing (asafoetida)
    2 teaspoons brown mustard seeds
    1 teaspoon ghee or oil

Bring the water to boil in a saucepan. Put the lentils in a shallow dish and pick through them to remove any tiny stones that might be hiding there. Wash the lentils in several changes of cool water until water runs clear. Pour them into the boiling water. Bring back to a boil, lower heat to simmer, and add the salt, ghee, and Vata Churna. Or heat the spices in ghee and add to the cooking lentils. Cover and simmer gently for 20 to 30 minutes, stirring occasionally.

When the lentils are tender and the dahl is a thick soup, fry the mustard seeds in oil or ghee until they just start to pop. It will make a swooshing sound as you add them to the dahl. Serve with a bowl of rice.

## Spiced Vegetable Curry

The secret of this mixed vegetable curry with its many subtle flavors is to prepare the ingredients in two separate pans with different spice combinations, then mix everything together at the end for rich and varied flavors that are delightfully discovered while eating. To receive the full benefit of a certain taste, it is necessary to experience it as clearly as possible. That's why AyurVeda recommends preparing certain taste and quality combinations separately, then combining them before serving.

All the ingredients are washed, peeled, chopped, ground, and so forth before beginning to cook. A labor-saving tip is to use Kapha Churna, a special blend of herbs and spices that helps balance Kapha dosha and adds a reasonable amount of spiciness at the same time. Select fresh, seasonally available vegetables. If you omit those vegetables not available that are listed in this recipe, be sure to substitute others in the correct quantity to make up the total amount called for. Although fresh vegetables are always the best choice, buying good quality fresh tomatoes, peas, and other summer favorites might not be practical in winter. The occasional use—once every week or two—of canned or frozen ingredients is all right as long as they make up a small part of the recipe.

This Spiced Vegetable Curry decreases Kapha and Vata, and increases Pitta somewhat. It makes a good side dish for Pitta when served as part of a meal with other Pitta-reducing selections. The predominant tastes are pungent, sour, sweet, slightly bitter, and astringent with hot, oily qualities. This combination makes it a good main dish anytime for those following a Kapha-reducing diet.

Serves 6 to 8

Prepare Vegetables:

   4 medium carrots, sliced
   4 small zucchini, sliced thin
   1 1/2 cups green beans, cut in 1/2- inch pieces
   1/2 cup peas, fresh or frozen
   1 small cauliflower, broken into flowerets
   1 small eggplant, peeled and diced
   3 to 4 medium tomatoes, skinned and diced
          or
   1 18-ounce can peeled tomatoes, chopped in blender or food processor

For the Curry:

    3 tablespoons ghee
    1 tablespoon Kapha Churna, or more to taste
    1 teaspoon salt
    1/2 cup water, or more as needed
    3 tablespoons olive oil, or other cooking oil
    1 teaspoon turmeric
    3/4 teaspoon ground cumin

In a Large Pot:

Heat 3 tablespoons ghee over moderate heat. Add Kapha Churna, stir briefly, then add carrots and zucchini slices. Turn heat to low and stir until well-coated with ghee. Cover and allow to simmer for 3 minutes. Add green beans, peas, salt, and 1/2 cup water. Cover and continue simmering on low while preparing the other ingredients.

In a Frying Pan or Large Wok:

Heat 2 tablespoons oil over moderately high heat. Add turmeric and cumin. Mix well together for about 30 seconds, then stir in cauliflower. Stir fry about 2 minutes or until cauliflower is evenly coated and bright gold. Push cauliflower to the sides of the pan and add 1 tablespoon of oil to the center. When it is hot stir in eggplant. Cook 1 minute. Then mix tomatoes in with the eggplant and cauliflower. Stir until eveything is well blended. It should become very liquid, like a tomato sauce. If not, add water gradually. Cover and turn heat to low and simmer 3 to 4 minutes.

  About 10 minutes before serving stir the tomato mixture into the large pot. Mix gently and simmer on low. Serve with rice.

Note: If any curry is left after the meal, save it until evening and heat it by frying in hot oil. Then stuff it in folded chapatis, tortillas, or pita bread. Serve these with a tossed salad for a light meal.

## Sweet Summer Curry

Curries are sometimes thought of fiery dishes that must be followed by lots of cool drinks and yogurt. Not this one. It is sweet and unctuous, astringent, warm, heavy, and a little salty. It is a good main dish for Pitta and Vata. Kapha can eat very moderately of this curry. The more pungent dishes suit Kapha better. By increasing the spinach and decreasing the raisins, grapes, and potatoes this sweet curry is a good side dish for Kapha types. When using sprouted lentils for frying, soak them in warm water, cover, and allow to sit overnight or just long enough for the sprouts to begin coming out. The lentil has its greatest nutritional value at this point, rather than when it is allowed to grow a long root. Wash the sprouted lentils well in cool water before using.

Serves 4 to 6 generously

Prepare Fried-Spiced Potatoes and allow them to steam while you cook the fruits and vegetables.

## Fried-Spiced Potatoes

1/4 cup light oil, safflower or sunflower
1/2 teaspoon nutmeg
1/2 teaspoon ground cardamom
1/2 teaspoon coriander
4 medium red skinned potatoes, scrubbed and diced
1/2 teaspoon salt
1/2 cup warm water

In a heavy frying pan heat oil over medium high heat. Add nutmeg, cardamom, and coriander. Stir in potatoes. When they are coated with oil and spices sprinkle salt. Fry over moderate heat, stirring frequently, for 10 minutes. Pour in water, cover, and simmer on low heat for 5 minutes. Turn off heat and leave covered until ready to combine with remaining ingredients.

To Curry Vegetables and Fruits:

4 to 6 tablespoons ghee
1/2 teaspoon brown mustard seeds (or poppy seeds for Pitta)
2 tablespoons Pitta Churna
1 cup sprouted whole urad lentils (Indian black gram)
2 apples, peeled and diced
2 medium yellow summer squash, diced
3/4 teaspoon salt
1/2 cup raisins
1/2 cup seedless grapes, green or red
1 cup  sweet fruit juice: pineapple, coconut, papaya (not for Pitta),
   mango, or white grape
3/4 cup toasted coconut
1/2 cup spinach, washed and chopped

In a large frying pan or wok heat 2 tablespoons ghee over medium high heat. Add mustard seeds (or poppy seeds). When seeds begin to pop add Pitta Churna. Stir for 1 minute. Add sprouts. Cook 2 to 3 minutes, stirring frequently. Push the sprouts to the sides of the pan and add 2 more table-spoons of ghee in the center. When  ghee is hot, add chopped apples  and squash. Stir in salt. Cook, stirring gently, for 3 to 4 minutes, then mix together with the sprouts. Add raisins, grapes, and fruit juice. Cover and simmer on low for 10 minutes. Gently toss in fried potatoes and mix well.

Stir in 1/2 cup toasted coconut. Reserve 1/4 cup for garnish. Spread spinach evenly on top and sprinkle with remaining coconut. Cover. Turn off heat and let steam for 10 minutes. Serve on a platter of Saffron Rice or plain rice for Pitta dieters in hot weather.

## Toasted Coconut

Heat 2 tablespoons ghee in a small pan over moderate heat. Add coconut and toss well to coat.  Heat slowly, stirring constantly until light brown. Remove from heat and set aside.

## About Raita

Raita is a yogurt-based side dish that serves as a sour, cold, refreshing foil to a spicy meal. As part of a whole meal and when eaten in small amounts, it is good for everyone. In large quantities it increases Pitta and Kapha. Finely shredded carrots or radishes make a colorful raita, but almost any minced or shredded raw vegetable mixed with yogurt qualifies as raita.

## Raita

1 to 2 cups plain yogurt
1/4 teaspoon cumin, freshly roasted and ground

Stir yogurt into a serving bowl. Sprinkle most of the cumin on top and stir in. Sprinkle the rest on top. Cover and refrigerate 30 minutes before serving.

## Tomato and Cucumber Raita

A refreshing raita that adds sour and slightly salty tastes to the meal, and cold, heavy qualities.

Makes 2 cups

1 small cucumber, peeled, seeded, and chopped
1/2 teaspoon salt
2 cups plain yogurt
1 medium tomato, skinned and chopped
1/2 teaspoon cumin seeds, roasted and ground

Mix cucumber and salt together in a small glass or stainless steel bowl. Set aside for about 15 minutes to drain the liquid out of the cucumber. Mix yogurt and tomato together in a serving bowl. Squeeze the juice from the cucumber until it feels dry and add it to the yogurt. Discard the juice. Stir in 1/4 teaspoon cumin. Sprinkle the rest on top. Cover tightly and refrigerate 30 minutes to an hour before serving.

## About Chutneys And Other Condiments

It is probably easier to eat AyurVedically balanced meals dining on the Indian cuisine than any other. Since India is "home of the Vedas" one would expect this to be so. A feast in the Indian style includes quite an array of small dishes brimming with stewed fruits, nuts, pickles, and vegetables that offer a splendid variety of tastes and qualities to choose from. These chutneys and other Indian condiments, the jewels of the Indian cuisine, make any good meal even more interesting. A chutney may contain only one taste or all the tastes needed to balanced the meal. And they can be served effectively at nearly any meal, not just Indian ones.

Varied condiments give each person a chance to select and balance the different tastes according to his needs. Although there are several recipes for chutneys and condiments in this sample menu, only a few are actually served at each meal. For a simple dinner one or two chutneys are probably enough.

## Kinds Of Chutneys

There are three kinds of chutneys: fresh, cooked, and preserved. Preserved chutneys keep on the kitchen shelf for several months. Usually these are the imported kinds that are preserved in oil, which AyurVeda considers a healthful way of food preserving.

Cooked chutneys keep well in the refrigerator for one or two months. They are made with large amounts of sugar, chilies, salt, oil, or vinegar, which all have preserving qualities.

Fresh chutneys are only used for one day. These "daily" chutneys are usually made in small amounts. If any fresh chutney is left at the end of the noon meal it can be fried in ghee or oil as the base for sautéed vegetables or soup at the next meal. Otherwise discard it.

## Fresh Green Chutney

This is a refresh ing "daily" chutney that should not be kept as a leftover into the next day. It is astringent, bitter, pungent, a little sweet, and salty. A little eaten with a meal is good for all doshas and helps with digestion. If making this for a small group, prepare only half the recipe.

Makes 1 cup or enough for a feast

> 1 cup chopped fresh parsley, coriander leaves, and/or spinach
> 1 teaspoon salt
> 1 lemon or lime, juiced
> 1 teaspoon cayenne, or less, to taste
> 1/4 cup water
> 1/4 cup dried coconut

Put all ingredients in a blender or food processor with a steel blade. Blend on low speed. Put in serving dish and set aside for 1 to 2 hours before serving.

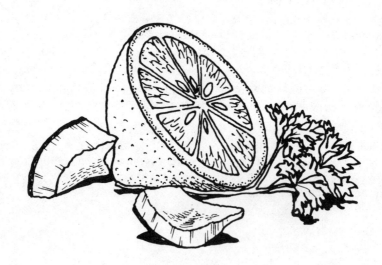

## Apple-Raisin Chutney

This chutney, and all chutneys in this Indian menu, is good in moderation for all doshas when they are served as part of a meal. This recipe is especially nourishing for Vata dosha. The addition of Kapha Churna gives a pungent taste making it better for Kapha types. It is sweet, pungent, hot, and a little astringent. It helps maintain the appetite when eaten throughout the meal.

Apple-Raisin Chutney can be saved in capped, sterilized jars in the refrigerator for a month. By reducing the Kapha Churna to one teaspoon, this recipe makes a tasty turnover filling for a Vata and Pitta dessert.

Makes 2 1/2 cups

    2 cups apples, peeled and chopped
    1/2 cup water
    1 teaspoon nutmeg
    1/4 teaspoon cloves
    3 to 4 tablespoons white sugar
    1/4 cup brown sugar
    2 tablespoons Kapha Churna
    1 cup raisins

Put the apples in a large pan. Add the other ingredients and cook over moderate heat, adding more water 1/4 cup at a time to keep chutney from drying out. Stir frequently until apples are tender and transparent, about 30 minutes. Stir well to blend into a sauce. Cool and serve. Store in refrigerator.

## Coconut Chutney

When served as an appetizer or condiment with the meal this rich, golden chutney adds sweet, pungent, oily, heavy properties to the meal.

Makes about 1 1/2 cups

1 tablespoon ghee
3/4 teaspoon cayenne
1/4 cup milk or cream
1 to 2 tablespoons sugar, to taste
1/8 teaspoon allspice
1/8 to 1/4 teaspoon saffron, crushed
1/4 cup raisins
1 cup coconut (finely chopped is best, but flaked will do)

Heat ghee over medium high heat in a small saucepan or frying pan. Then add cayenne and stir about one minute. Stir in milk, sugar, allspice, and crumbled saffron threads. Bring to a boil, stirring often. Milk should begin turning golden yellow. Reduce heat to simmer. Stir in raisins and 1 cup coconut. Beat well as mixture leaves sides of the pan. If it is too liquid, add more coconut, a tablespoon at a time, until the mixture is just moist but not wet. Serve in a small bowl.

## Fresh Ginger Lemon Chutney

A good appetizer for Vata and Kapha, this chutney is a pleasant accompaniment to many meals besides Indian ones. Left over, this chutney is especially delicious fried with vegetables, or tossed with hot rice or other cooked grains.

Makes 1/2 cup

> 1 lemon
> 1/4 pound fresh ginger, peeled
> 1/2 teaspoon salt
> 1/2 teaspoon sugar, optional

Peel the lemon with a vegetable peeler or zester. Then mince or chop the peel very fine. Squeeze lemon juice into a small cup. Chop ginger into small chunks in a blender or food processor for 30 seconds. Measure 1/2 cup ginger and leave it in the blender container. Add lemon peel, 1/2 teaspoon lemon juice, salt, and sugar. Blend again for 30 seconds or until the mixture looks soft and tan. Serve in a tiny bowl or dish. It keeps one day.

## Kashmiri Mint Chutney

An authentic and most exotic way to make this fresh chutney is by collecting the wild mint that grows on the hillsides of Sonmarg, "the Sun Meadow," an alpine meadow at 10,000 feet in Kashmir. But any fresh mint can be substituted until you can get the real thing. As with other chutneys, mint chutney is good for all doshas as part of a balanced meal, especially for Kapha and Pitta. The tastes in this chutney are astringent, sour, pungent, slightly sweet, and bitter.

Makes 1 cup

> 2/3 cup fresh mint leaves, washed, dried, minced
> 1/4 cup ground walnuts
> 1 teaspoon yogurt
> 1/2 teaspoon turmeric

Mix minced mint leaves and walnuts together. In a small cup stir yogurt and tumeric together, then blend with mint. Cover and allow to sit for 30 minutes before serving.

## Tomato Chutney

Everyone can eat some of this chutney as part of a balanced meal, but it increases Pitta dosha if eaten in any more than a small quantity. It has sour, pungent, astringent, sweet, salty, oily, and slightly bitter properties. This cooked chutney keeps well for two weeks tightly covered in the refrigerator.

Makes 2 cups

To Prepare Spices:

> 1 tablespoon ghee
> 1 teaspoon brown mustard seeds
> 1/2 teaspoon fenugreek, ground
> 1 teaspoon cumin seeds, dry roasted and ground
> 1 teaspoon coriander, ground
> 1 teaspoon freshly grated ginger
> > or
> > 3/4 teaspoon ground ginger
> 1/2 teaspoon turmeric

Heat ghee in a heavy pot over moderate heat. Add mustard seeds and when they start to pop stir in the other spices. Fry for one minute, stirring constantly.

For the Tomato Mixture:

> 10 medium tomatoes, peeled and mashed
> 1 teaspoon salt
> 1/4 teaspoon sweet paprika (optional)
> 1 tablespoon brown sugar, or to taste
> 1 teaspoon lemon juice

Add the tomatoes to the spices, then stir in the remaining ingredients. Turn to simmer and heat for 10 to 15 minutes, stirring until everything is thoroughly blended. Cover and allow to cook on low for another 10 minutes. Cool and serve.

## Quick Condiments

Here are a few easy condiments that add taste, texture, color and more variety to an Indian dinner. Small bowls and dishes of chutneys and condiments make the meal both interesting to the eye and the palate.

## Spiced Cashew Nuts

A few of these sweet, oily, slightly heavy nuts are good for Vata and Pitta, and increase Kapha, especially if they are eaten in excess (easy to do). They keep well on the kitchen shelf or in the refrigerator.

Makes 1 cup

> 1 1/2 tablespoons ghee
> 1 cup unsalted cashew nuts, broken in pieces
> 1/2 teaspoon of *one* of the following ground spices:
>     cardamom, ginger, nutmeg, cinnamon, or coriander

Heat ghee in a small pan over moderate heat. Sprinkle in nuts and spice. Stir frequently until nuts are toasty brown. Serve in a small bowl. If saved for another meal, reheat briefly over a low flame.

## Toasted Coconut Condiment

Serve a small dish of coconut plain or toasted so it can be sprinkled over some favorite curry on the dinner plate. If toasted coconut is served as a condiment, do not serve another coconut chutney as well. A little of the sweet, heavy and oily properties of coconut go a long way. They are good for Vata and Pitta, and increase Kapha.

> 1 tablespoon ghee
> 1/2 to 2/3 cup flaked coconut
> 1/4 teaspoon saffron, drumbled (optional)

Heat ghee in a small pan over low heat. Toss in coconut and stir frequently until it is just brown on the tips. Put in serving dish immediately.

## Lemon And Lime Wedges

Wedged lemons and limes are good to serve at any main meal. They add both color and a sour taste, help clear the palate when eaten with the heavier parts of the dinner, and in small qualtities, they aid digestion. Cut washed lemons and limes in narrow wedges and arrange in alternating colors on a small plate.

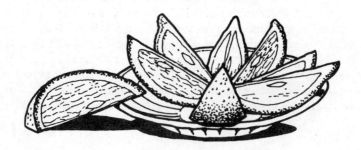

## Puris and Chapatis

Typical Indian main dishes are served with fried unleavened breads used for "pushing" the food and sopping up the delectable juices. Puris and Chapatis, the most frequently eaten of these breads, are good for everyone, although the sweet and heavy qualities can increase Kapha if too many are eaten. While the ingredients are identical, Chapatis are fried on a hot griddle and Puris, puffy breads, are deep fried in oil.

Makes 15 to 20 Puris or 10 Chapatis

    1 1/2 cups whole wheat flour
    1/2 cup white flour
    1/2 teaspoon salt
    1 tablespoon ghee
    3/4 cup hot water
    3 to 4 cups oil for frying Puris

In a large bowl stir flours and salt together. Rub in ghee with fingertips until it is evenly combined with flour. Add water and stir into a dough. Add a little more water by teaspoons, if needed, to completely blend all the flour. Knead for 4 or 5 minutes in the bowl. Cover with plastic wrap and allow to rest 1 or 2 hours. The consistency of workable dough should be pliable and firm, but not sticky.

To Make Puris:

Pinch off 1-inch balls of douch, roll in a little flour, then gently roll out on a wooden surface with a rolling pin. Roll in one direction only. Turn the dough over and roll in the opposite direction until it is 4 to 5 inches across and about as thin as a penny, not thinner. Heat oil in a deep, heavy pan or wok over moderately high heat. When oil is hot gently ease a Puri in so it goes under the surface to the bottom of the pan. When it rises to the top use a pair of tongs and gently push it back under the oil. It should blow up like a balloon. Turn it over in the oil and cook 30 seconds more. Remove and drain on paper towels. Cook each Puri separately and drain.

To Make Chapatis:

Pinch off 2-inch pieces of dough. Roll out evenly and fry on hot greased griddle or heavy skillet for about 30 seconds on each side. Serve immediately.

## Laddu
## (Cashew Nut Balls)

Laddus are ball-shaped sweets something between cookies and candy. Like most Indian desserts they are very sweet and nourishing. This dessert is good for Vata and Pitta, and in small smounts good for Kapha, too. They make a sweet, unctuous, slightly heavy, and satisfying end to an Indian meal.

Makes 1 1/2 dozen

1 teaspoon ghee
3 tablespoons cashews
4 tablespoons ghee
1 cup besan (chickpea) flour, from Asian or natural food store, or substitute whole wheat flour
6 green cardamom pods, seeded and ground
    or
  1/2 teaspoon fresh ground cardamom
1 cup brown sugar

Melt teaspoon ghee in a small pan over low heat. Add nuts and fry until lightly toasted. Remove from heat and chop fine in nut grinder. Set aside.

In a large skillet or heavy pan heat 4 tablespoons ghee. Add besan and cook over low heat, stirring frequently until golden. Watch carefully not to allow the flour to get too dark. Remove from heat and add the nuts and other ingredients, stirring well. The dough will leave the sides of the pan and be thick when well mixed. Cool until it can be handled, about 30 minutes. Roll each laddu into a small ball, smaller than a golf ball. Rub hands with ghee if dough sticks too much.

Arrange on a plate as they are rolled and set aside at least an hour, or until they are hard, before serving.

Store in a tightly sealed container.

## Fragrantly Spiced Lassi

Lassi, a yogurt-based drink traditionally served at the end of an Indian meal, is good for everyone to drink except late at night or in cold weather. The usual recipe for Lassi is simply yogurt thinned with water to taste. The more elaborate Fragrantly Spiced Lassi is served at dinner parties or special occasions. No matter what kind you make it should be served at the end of the meal rather than as an accompanying beverage. If taken in large amounts Lassi increases Pitta and Kapha. One cup per person is sufficient.

Makes 1 quart

    1 cup plain yogurt
    1/2 cup white sugar, or to taste
    3 cups cold water
    1 green cardamom pod, husked and seeded
           or
     1/4 teaspoon ground caramom
    Pinch of saffron, crumbled
    1/8 teaspoon nutmeg
    1 teaspoon rosewater

Mix yogurt and water together in a bowl, beating until smooth. Add water and spices. Stir well, cover, and refrigerate 2 to 4 hours. Just before serving stir in rosewater.

## A FRENCH MENU

POTAGE PRINTANIER
(Sweet, Salty, Slightly Astringent, Light)

PETIT POIS BRAISE LAITUE
(Sweet, Sour)

SIMPLE RICE PILAF
(Sweet, Salty, Light)

TOSSED GREEN SALAD
(Bitter, Astringent, Pungent)

FRENCH BREAD WITH SWEET BUTTER
(Sweet, Heavy)

PECHE CARDINAL
(Sweet, Heavy, Cold)

## Potage Printanier

This is a light, flavorful potato soup in the French style. It takes less than an hour to make and your guests will think it took much longer. Within the context of the whole menu this soup is nourishing for everyone. A steaming bowl of Potage Printanier, a tossed green salad, and a slice of lightly buttered bread makes a good light supper for Kapha types. Tastes in this recipe are sweet, salty, and a little astringent.

Serves 8

2 tablespoons butter or ghee
1 green pepper, chopped
1 1/2 quarts hot water
2 potatoes, pared, quartered, sliced thin
2 carrots, sliced
1/4 cup white rice
6 stalks asparagus, cut in 1/2-inch pieces
1/2 pound spinach, washed and chopped
1 cup light cream
Ground pepper to taste

Melt butter or ghee in a large pot. Add green pepper and sauté until soft. Add water, potatoes, and carrot. Bring to a boil, then reduce to simmer for 15 minutes, stirring occasionally. Add the rice and asparagus. Cover and simmer over very low heat for 25 minutes. Remove the cover and stir in the spinach. Simmer for another 10 minutes. Finally, just before serving add the light cream and just heat through, but do not boil.

## For weight watchers and Kapha in spring time:

Decrease to 1 potato, 1/2 cup cream mixed with 1/2 cup water or one cup of skim milk, and 1 tablespoon of butter or ghee.

## Pois Braise Laitue
## (Peas Braised with Lettuce)

This dish is a delightful blend of sweet and sour tastes. It combines consistency with the refreshing lightness of spring vegetables and makes a satisfying entree served with Rice Pilaf. The recipe has a neutral effect on Vata and Pitta doshas and increases Kapha slightly.

Serves 4 to 6

1 firm Boston lettuce
3 sprigs each:
        parsley
        thyme
        marjoram
2 tablespoons butter
1 pepper—red bell or pimento, diced or chopped
2 cups fresh peas
1 cup chopped spinach
1/2 cup water
1/2 teaspoon salt
1/2 teaspoon sugar

Wash lettuce and cut into 4 to 6 wedges. Tie each wedge together with cotton string to keep its shape. Tie herb sprigs together. In a heavy 3-quart saucepan put all the ingredients except 2 tablespoons of butter. Bring to a boil over moderate heat, tossing lightly. Cover the pan and cook over low heat for 30 minutes, stirring frequently until vegetables are tender and the liquid is cooked away. Remove the herbs and the strings from the lettuce wedges. Add 2 tablespoons butter, toss, and serve on a bed of rice.

Note: Sugar and butter can be reduced by half for those watching their weight.

## Simple Rice Pilaf

This simple dish to make adds sweet and salty tastes to the meal.  It is best served with steamed or sautéed vegetables.

Makes about 2 cups

>    3 tablespoons ghee or butter
>    1 stalk celery, chopped
>    1 cup white rice
>    1/2 teaspoon basil, crushed,
>                    or
>      1 teaspoon fresh basil, chopped
>    1 tablespoon parsley, chopped
>    1/2 teaspoon salt
>    1/2 teaspoon  pepper, or to taste
>    2  cups water

Melt ghee in a 2-quart saucepan and sauté celery. Add rice and cook about one minute until rice is transparent.  Ghee should just cover rice.  Add basil, parsley, salt, and pepper.  Then add water.  Bring to boil, reduce to low heat, and simmer covered tightly for about 20 minutes or until all the water is absorbed.  Fluff and serve.

For Pitta: Omit the basil and increase the parsley to taste.

## French Bread

The taste and crunchy texture is authentically French. This bread, like most plain wheat flour breads, is sweet and good for general nutrition. Eaten in moderation it reduces Vata and Kapha, and is neutral for Pitta. It's best to always eat bread *with* butter for ease of digestion. Vegetables and bread compliment each other by being most efficiently assimilated when eaten during the same course of the meal.

Makes 2 to 3 loaves

    2 packages yeast
    3 cups tepid water
    7 1/2 cups unbleached bread flour
    4 teaspoons salt

In a small bowl dissolve the yeast in warm water. In a large bowl mix flour and salt together. Form a well and with a wooden spoon incorporate water and yeast into the flour. Work the flour into a ball by hand, and then transfer to a floured work surface. The dough will feel tacky. Knead dough for about 10 minutes, adding small amounts of flour as necessary. Occasionally throw dough on the work surface. After 10 minutes it will become elastic, but will remain a bit sticky. Grease a large bowl and place dough in it. Cover tightly with plastic wrap. Set in a warm place and allow to double in volume. This will take about 1 1/2 to 2 hours. Punch down, cover, and let rise again. Turn out on a floured surface and knead briefly. Divide into as many loaves as desired. If you are using a French baguette pan, divide the dough into thirds, and make 2 baguettes and 1 oval loaf. Otherwise, two nicely rounded loaves can be made. Place the loaves, covered lightly with a towel, in a warm place and let rise to double volume.

Preheat oven to 425°.

Place a shallow pan of water on the lowest oven shelf. Before putting loaves in oven, slash tops diagonally with razor blade or very sharp knife point. Then spray the loaves with water before placing in oven. Bake on preheated baking tile or on baking sheets sprinkled with a little cornmeal. During the first 18 minutes of baking, open the oven door and spray the loaves with water several times. This will make them very crispy. Remove the pan of water and finish baking until golden brown. Total baking time is 25-30 minutes. Cool on rack.

## Peche Cardinal

The brilliant red and gold colors of this dessert announce an impressive conclusion to the French dinner. It is a combination of sweet tastes good for both Vata and Pitta. Kapha types should eliminate the Chantilly cream and eat lightly of this dish.

Serves 6

> 4 cups water
> 1 1/2 cups sugar
> 6 large peaches, peeled, halved, and pitted
> 2 tablespoons vanilla

In a heavy saucepan bring water and sugar to a boil over high heat, stirring constantly until sugar dissolves. Boil 3 minutes, then reduce heat. Add peaches and vanilla. Simmer 15 minutes or until barely tender when tested with a fork. Cover and refrigerate while preparing other ingredients.

For the Cardinal Sauce:

> 2 10-ounce packages frozen raspberries, or 2 cups fresh raspberries
> 2 tablespoons fine granulated or confectioners sugar

Drain raspberries in a sieve and purée with a wooden spoon. Discard seeds and pulp. Stir sugar into the raspberry juice and refrigerate in tightly covered container.

Cream Chantilly:

> 1/2 cup heavy cream, chilled
> 1 1/2 tablespoons sugar, fine granulated or confectioners
> 2 teaspoons vanilla

Whip cream until thick. Sprinkle in sugar and vanilla. Continue beating until it is firm enough to hold soft peaks. To serve: Arrange peaches halves in individual dishes or on a platter. Spoon Cardinal Sauce over each peach. Top with Cream Chantilly. Use the leftover peach cooking syrup for poaching other fruit, if desired.

## ITALIAN MENU

CHEESE CRACKERS AND ITALIAN CHEESES
(Salty, Sweet, Slightly Pungent, Sour, Oily)

PASTA AND GREEN SAUCE
(Sweet, Salty, OIly, Heavy)

FAGIOLONI IN UMIDO VOLPONI
(Sweet, Salty)

SPINACH AND CHICORY SALAD
(Bitter, Astringent, Pungent, Light, Hot)

MACEDONIA DI FRUITA
(Sweet, Cold, Heavy)

ITALIAN HAZELNUT COOKIES
(Sweet, Bitter, Astringent, Dry)

## Cheese Crackers

These appetizers are more like soft little biscuits than crackers. Traditionally they are served warm with a selection of Italian cheeses, such as Parmesan, fontini, and mozzarella. Pitta should eat lightly from the cheese tray. Whether eaten by themselves, or with soup, these little cheese crackers add a salty taste that is slightly pungent, and sweet. Eating them reduces Vata, is neutral for Pitta, and increases Kapha.

Serves 6 generously

1 cup flour
1/2 teaspoon salt
1/2 teaspoon paprika
Coarsely ground black pepper to taste
1/2 cup butter
1 cup grated cheese, Parmesan, Romano, or cheddar in combination
2 tablespoons heavy cream
1/2 tablespoon heavy cream for glaze

Preheat oven to 325°.

Stir the flour together with the salt, paprika, and pepper. With a pastry cutter or the steel knife of a food processor, cut the butter in until it is mealy. Stir in heavy cream. When you have a smooth dough, chill it for about an hour. Roll out the dough on a floured surface to a thickness of about 1/4 inch. Cut into strips 1/2 inch by 1 1/2 inches. Brush with the cream and arrange on ungreased baking sheets. Bake for 12 to 14 minutes until puffy and a little brown.

## Pasta and Green Sauce

The green herbs make this sauce a flavorful accompaniment to spaghetti or linguini. When served with pasta this dish decreases Vata, is neutral for Pitta, and increases Kapha. Kapha can eat more of this as a main dish if cooked barley is substituted for the pasta. Parmesan cheese can be used by both Vata and Kapha. The combined qualities of this recipe are sweet, salty, oily, and heavy.

Serves 4 to 6

    1 cup minced parsley
    3/4 cup minced fresh basil or 1/2 cup dried crushed basil
    1 teaspoon salt
    1/2 cup chopped nuts—pine nuts are best
    1/2 cup olive oil
    Grated parmesan cheese, optional

Grind herbs, salt, and nuts in mortar and pestle, or chop in a food processor with a steel blade. Add the oil and combine until smooth. This makes about 1 1/2 cups of simple "pesto."

Cook spaghetti or other pasta according to package directions. Drain and toss with green sauce.

## Green Beans in Tomato Sauce
## (Fagioloni in Umido Volponi)

A delicious main dish this has properly balanced tastes and qualities that reduce all doshas. It is pleasantly sweet and salty. The green beans must be very well cooked to reduce Vata.

Serves 4

1 pound fresh green beans
1 pound ripe tomatoes, or a 14-ounce can of tomatoes, chopped
2 tablespoons olive oil or vegetable oil
1/2 teaspoon each of oregano, thyme, and basil
Salt and pepper to taste

Wash, de-string, and cut beans into 1-inch pieces. Blanch and peel fresh tomatoes, then chop. Heat the oil in a 2-quart saucepan. Add beans, tomatoes, and crushed herbs. Stir a few times, then add salt and pepper to taste. Cover and simmer over low heat for about 45 minutes, until the beans are quite tender and the tomatoes saucy. If the sauce starts to stick, add a little water during cooking. Serve hot with pasta.

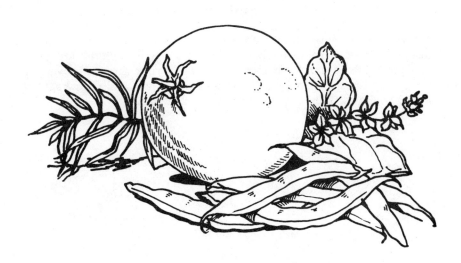

## Spinach and Chicory Salad

The bitter, astringent, slightly pungent, light, hot, and dry properties of this salad are especially balancing for a Kapha diet. It is also a good salad to prepare when serving people with varied dietary needs. If the meal consists of several heavy or sweet dishes, then those following a Kapha diet can help themselves to a large amount of this healthy salad. Vata and Pitta types would eat smaller portions.

Serves 4

1/4 cup basic vinaigrette dressing
1 teaspoon dry mustard
1/4 teaspoon nutmeg
2 teaspoons Kapha Churna
      or
1 teaspoon coarsely ground black pepper
1/2 teaspoon ground fenugreek
1/4 teaspoon ground cumin
1/4 teaspoon ground coriander
2 cups spinach, washed and torn into bite-size pieces
1 small head chicory—radicchio type
1/2 cup red cabbage, thinly shredded
3 to 4 red radishes, thinly sliced
3 tablespoons blanched, slivered almonds, optional

Mix vinaigrette, mustard, and Kapha Churna together. If a spice blend is used instead of the Churna, then mix the dry spices together before adding to the vinaigrette. Place spinach in a serving bowl and pour vinaigrette over. Toss well. Add remaining veegetables. Toss again, cover, and refrigerate for at least 30 minutes. Before serving sprinkle with almonds.

## Macedonia di Fruita

All the fruits in this salad are good for the all doshas when eaten as a part of a meal, but it would not be good for Kapha as a separate meal. For the culinary artist these fruits are like colors on a palette waiting to be made into something spectacular. When prepared in a grand manner this dish can be used as an impressive centerpiece for a buffet dessert.

Servess 8 to 10

      4 apples, sweet, not tart
      3 sweet oranges
      1 large cantaloupe, balls or cubes
      2 cups cubed watermelon
      1 medium honeydew melon, balls or cubes
                    or
         Any other melon varieties in season
      8 to 12 Calmyrna figs
      8 to 10 small bunches unsprayed grapes, red, green, and deep purple
      10 to 12 pitted dates
      Other seasonal fruits of choice

Core and thickly slice the apples. Wash the oranges thoroughly and slice with their skins on, or peel and section. Cube or ball the melons. Clip the washed grapes into individual bunches. Arrange the fruits in little groups of 8 to 10 with some of every fruit in each group. Individual servings can be made ahead of time.

## Italian Hazelnut Cookies

These delicate cookies are sweet, bitter, astringent, dry, and good for all doshas. When made with both wheat and barley flour they are best for Kapha. If you don't have barley flour on hand, use all white flour. These cookies pack well to send as gifts. The anise flavor develops best when they are stored in a sealed container for a day or two.

Makes 2 1/2 dozen

> 1 cup butter (1/2 pound), softened at room temperature
> 1/4 cup sugar
> 2 teaspoons anise extract
> > or
> 3 teaspoons ground anise seeds
> 1/2 cup barley flour
> 1 1/2 cups unbleached white flour
> > or
> 2 cups unbleached white flour
> 1/4 teaspoon salt
> 3/4 cup finely ground hazelnuts (or pecans)
> 1/2 cup powdered sugar

Preheat oven to 300°.

Cream butter and sugar together. Mix in anise extract or ground seeds. Measure dry ingredients in a separate bowl and mix together thoroughly. Stir in nuts, then add dry iingredients to the butter mixture.

Shape into balls or 2 x 2 1/2-inch crescents. Roll in powdered sugar. Bake on ungreased cookie sheets in the center of the oven until faintly brown, about 12 minutes. (Gently turn one cookie over to test for color.) When cool roll again in powdered sugar.

# AMERICAN PICNIC MENU

TOFU NUT BURGERS
with CONDIMENTS
(Sweet, Heavy)

OVEN BAKED FRENCH FRIES
(Sweet, Oily, Heavy)

CONFETTI RICE SALAD
(Sweet, Slightly Bitter, Pungent, Sour, Cold, Light)

TOSSED GREEN SALAD
(Bitter, Astringent, Pungent,Light)

WATERMELON
(Sweet, Cold)

SUPER CHOCOLATE BROWNIES
(Bitter, Sweet, Astringent, Slightly Salty)

AMERICAN APPLE PIE
(Sweet, Heavy)

WATERMELON-STRAWBERRY PUNCH
(Sweet, Cold)

## Tofu Nut Burgers

A good main dish that is both sweet and nourishing, tofu nut burgers have a tonic (heathfully nourishing) effect. They are a body-building food that decreases Vata, is neutral for Pitta, and increases Kapha. When eaten with the usual selection of condiments—pickles, olives, mustard, catsup, and so forth—they are more easily digested. Choose from condiments according to taste.

Makes 8 burgers

    1 pound tofu
    2 cups cooked brown rice
    1 cup ground nuts—medium grind
    3 tablespoons tamari, or to taste
    1 stalk of celery, chopped and sautéed

Preheat oven to 350°.

Combine tofu with 1 1/2 cups brown rice in a food processor, blending thoroughly. Add remaining ingredients, mix, and form into patties. Bake on greased baking sheet for 25 to 35 minutes. A nice brown crust will form on the outside but they will stay moist on the inside.

Serve hot, or save and reheat by putting in 350° oven for 5 minutes.

Tofu burgers can be baked at the same time as the Oven-Baked French Fries.

## Oven-Baked French Fries

French fries, a very popular American food that nearly everyone loves, are so heavy, oily, and fat increasing that Kapha should eat less of them. French fries decrease Vata and are neutral for Pitta. This oven method results in "fried" potatoes that are easier to digest and less oily.

1 potato per person
1/2 tablespoon butter per person
Salt and pepper to taste

Preheat oven to 350°.

Slice potatoes in long thin "frenched" shapes. Melt the butter and coat the potatoes. Arrange them on baking sheets 1 or 2 layers thick. Bake for at least 1 hour, turning the potatoes after about 30 minutes. They are done when they turn golden brown. For large amounts—more than 5 potatoes—baking may take longer.

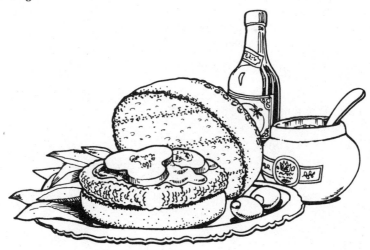

## Confetti Rice Salad

This is a pleasant summertime party salad that is especially good for Vata and Pitta. Kapha can eat this rice dish in moderation with a green leafy salad or separately as a light meal. This is a light, sweet, cold dish with some bitter, pungent, and sour tastes.

Makes 4 cups

2 1/2 cups cooked rice
1/2 yellow pepper, chopped
1/2 sweet red pepper chopped
1 full stalk celery (with leaves), chopped
4 tablespoons fresh parsley, chopped
1 1/2 tablespoons mixed fresh herbs of choice, such as basil, tarragon, summer savory, fennel,finely minced
5 tablespoons vinaigrette dressing
Salt and pepper to taste
Chopped parsely and paprika, optional garnish

While rice is still warm, toss with chopped vegetables, herbs, and dressing. Add salt and pepper to taste. Sprinkle on extra chopped parsley, or a little sweet paprika for color. Cover and chill for 2 or 3 hours.Serve on a bed of lettuce with wedges of tomato and sliced cucumber.

Suggestion: Sauté leftover rice salad in oil with vegetables for a satisfying side dish or light meal.

## Simple Vinaigrette Dressing

1/4 cup oil
1 tablespoon warm water
1 tablespoon vinegar
1/4 teaspoon salt

Place all ingredients in a small jar, cover tightly, and shake vigorously.

## Super Chocolate Brownies

Here is a rich chocolate brownie that is good for all doshas. The tastes are bitter, sweet, astringent, a little salty, and very delicious. The only thing wrong with these brownies is that you have to wait until they are completely cool to cut them. They are best made by hand and not with a food processor or electric mixer.

Makes 1 dozen brownies

> 1/2 cup butter or ghee
> 2 squares (2 ounces) unsweetened chocolate
> 1/3 cup flour
> 1 1/4 cups cool water
> 1/2 teaspoon salt
> 2 teaspoons vanilla
> 1/2 cup cocoa (best quality available)
> 2 cups flour
> 2 teaspoons baking powder
> 2 cups sugar
> 1 cup pecans or blanched almonds, coarsely chopped

Grease a 9 x 12-inch pan. Preheat oven to 350°.

For the Chocolate Mixture:

Melt the chocolate squares and butter together in a small heavy pan over low heat. Stir often. Set aside when melted and well-blended. In a small saucepan mix 1/3 cup flour with a little water to make a paste, then add the remaining water and cook over moderate heat, stirring constantly, until thickened, about 5 minutes. A few lumps are okay. Remove from heat and stir in salt, vanilla, and chocolate mixture. Cool while preparing the dry ingredients.

To Combine:

Measure dry ingredients into a large bowl. Stir well or sift together. Stir in sugar, liquid mixture, and then the nuts. Mix by hand until just blended, about one minute. The mixture will look very thick. Spread into the pan and bake for 25 to 30 minutes on the center oven rack. Brownies are done when they just start to leave the edges of the pan. For moist brownies, a knife inserted in the middle will not come out completely clean.

Remove from the oven and cool completely before cutting.

## American Apple Pie

What would an American picnic be without apple pie? This is a pleasantly spicy pie that is sweet and heavy. It decreases Vata and Pitta, and increases Kapha. By reducing the sugar and eliminating the nutmeg, Kapha can eat some of this pie. Or bake the Apple Pie without Sugar (recipe follows).

Pie crust for top and bottom of 9-inch pie

    3 to 4 cups apples—peeled and chopped
    1/2 cup sugar
    4 tablespoons brown sugar
    1 1/2 teaspoons cinnamon
    3/4 teaspoon cardamom
    1/4 teaspoon nutmeg
    Juice of one lemon

Preheat oven to 375°.

Mix all ingredients in a large bowl. Roll out half the pie crust dough on a floured surface. Carefully place it in a 9-inch pan without tearing. Heap apples toward the center of the pan. Roll out the rest of the dough and lay it on the apples. Seal the edges well and slit vents in the top to allow steam to escape. Bake on a cookie sheet for about one hour or until crust is nicely browned.

## Butter Pie Crust

Makes two 10-inch crusts

    3 cups flour
    1/4 teaspoon salt
    1 cup cold butter
    3 to 4 tablespoons ice water

Mix flour and salt together, then cut in butter with a pastry cutter, or chop with a knife until pieces are the size of currants or small peas. Add the ice water a tablespoon at a time, just until the dough will hold together to form a ball. Roll out on a floured surface. Try not to stretch or handle the dough more than necessary or it will become tough.

## Apple Pie Filling without Sugar

For those watching their weight but still wishing eat a good slice of American apple pie or a turnover, this is the filling to choose. A flour crust will add to its Kapha-increasing properties, but not very much. It reduces Vata and Pitta.

Pie crust for top and bottom of 9-inch pie

> 10 medium baking apples—Granny Smith, Jonathan, or Winesap
> Juice of one large lemon or two medium oranges
> 3/4 cup raisins
> 3 tablespoons cornstarch
> 2 tablespoons cinnamon

Preheat oven to 425°

Peel and slice apples very thinly. Add remaining ingredients and mix thoroughly. Roll out half the pie crust dough on a floured surface. Carefully place it in a 9-inch pan without tearing. Heap apples toward the center of the pan. Roll out the rest of the dough and lay it on the apples. Seal the edges well and cut slits in the top. Bake on a cookie sheet for 15 minutes at 425° then reduce to 350° and bake 45 minutes longer.

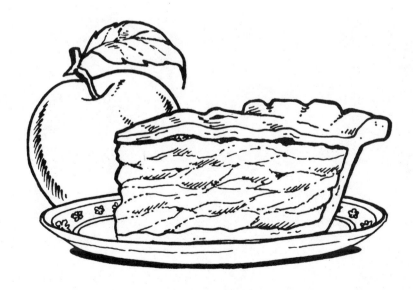

# Chapter 9

# Special Diets

## About Special Diets

The two special diets--weight loss and for new mother's--described in this chapter are recommended for normally active, healthy people. If you think you might need a restricted diet for a particular health problem such as diabetes, high blood pressure, serious overweight or underweight, high cholesterol, and so forth, consult your doctor or a Maharishi Ayur-Veda physician (listed at end of book). Following fads and radical diets as a basis for nutritional planning is foolish. If you want to eliminate or substantially increase anything in your diet, you should obtain qualified advice before you upset the natural balance of your physiology. Complete programs for normal health maintainence, weight loss, and maternity care are available through the Maharishi Ayur-Veda Health Centers.

*Eat correctly and live a normal human lifespan: 36,000 days and nights... a hundred years.*

- Dr. H.S. Kasture

## Weight Loss

Many times losing weight is simply a matter of carefully following rules for proper eating until they develop into good habits and eating a light diet. Suggestions for losing weight in this chapter are also good for balancing Kapha dosha. People with predominately Vata or Pitta constitutions should discuss eating a light diet with their physician before undertaking it. By following good eating practices maintaining normal weight is easier.

## Special Weight-Reducing Foods

Some foods are especially good for losing weight. Most of these are light and dry in quality. In a weight loss program favor foods with astringent, bitter, and pungent tastes.

189

## Grains

Eat barley once every day or every other day. It is light and astringent. Boiling it in seasoned water is good. By frying it in a little oil for two or three minutes or until it is lightly brown, barley becomes even lighter and less fattening. Barley water is a natural diuretic.

Other Kapha-reducing grains to include in a reducing diet are cornmeal, buckwheat, and rye. Avoid eating very much wheat and rice. Although it is all right to substitute a rice cake for a slice of bread because rice cakes are very light and dry.

## Spices, Teas, and Coffee

Increase the use of ginger, freshly grated is best, and black pepper, turmeric. During the day sip warm ginseng or other Kapha-reducing tea, such as Maharishi Ayur-Veda "Kapha Tea" or Celestial Seasonings "Emperor's Choice." Because black coffee and tea have a bitter taste, these are good for reducing Kapha.

## Salads and Fresh Vegetables

Bitter, astringent, light leafy greens, as well as such bitter-tasting steamed vegetables as Swiss chard, celery leaves, and unpeeled zucchini are part of an everyday weight loss diet.

## Balance

The proper balance of the six tastes and qualities is still important even when reducing weight. A healthy weight loss program includes variety from many food groups. Ninety-five percent of a main meal for weight loss should include Kapha-decreasing foods with bitter, pungent, and astringent tastes, and dry, light, and hot qualities predominating. The rest of the meal should be sweet, salty, sour, cold, heavy, and oily. Eat no Kapha-increasing desserts.

## Lots of Salads

As much as one half of the main meal can be a salad of lettuce, other leafy greens, and fresh herbs. Light, dry, pungent, bitter and astringent, salads have all the best qualities Kapha types and those reducing weight want most. But it is important to eat warm food, even as a sidedish, as well. A bowl of soup or steamed vegetables and cornbread, barley, or other light grains or a serving of spicy mixed vegetables and grain is best. Too much cold food will leave a dieter dissatisfied and hungry.

## Reduce Snacking

Do not eat in between meals. At the beginning of a weight loss diet, if you feel ravenously hungry (this feeling should subside in a day or two), *sit down* and eat a piece of dried fruit or nibble on a rice cake, just until you feel satisfied. Or sip some warm water or unsweetened tea.

*AyurVeda is dedicated
to all those who want to become
good eaters.*

-Dr. H. S. Kasture

## Good Eating Practices for Weight Loss

- Always sit down to eat.
- Eat only when hungry.
- Allow enough time to eat well.
- Never eat when upset.
- Pause in silence a minute or two before eating to balance the doshas, or say a brief prayer.
- Eat in a settled, serene atmosphere with pleasant table conversation, soft dinner music, or comfortable silence.
- Don't read, watch television, or drive a vehicle while eating.
- Don't talk on the telephone, listen to loud music, or receive visitors.
- Take comfortable bites of food and chew thoroughly.
- Sip water after every few bites of food.
- Eat the main meal at noonday.
- Eat very lightly in the evening and be finished before 8 p.m.
- Leave the table just satisfied, not full. If still hungry eat one or two more bites of food.
- Don't eat or drink anything but water or warm tea between meals.
- At the end of the meal sit and relax for 5 or 10 minutes.
- Don't drink anything for an hour after eating.
- Wait at least six hours before eating again.
- Eat freshly prepared food.
- Eat balanced meals that include some of the six tastes and six qualities.

## Light Meals and Fasting

Eating lightly once a week is restful to the digestive system. If you are in good health and it is comfortable, you might want to fast from all solid foods. Or follow any of the one-day fasts described in this chapter. If it is possible, eat very lightly or fast on the same day each week as part of your regular routine. Occasional light eating is salutary and purifying for the body. Before long you will look forward to that rest. Be sure, however, that the day you fast is a day of complete rest--one without work or strenuous mental or physical activity.

## Kinds of Fasts

A fast is just a rest, not an ascetic exercise. Even those with Pitta and Vata constitutions can benefit from a day of lighter eating, but a full fast from all food may not be comfortable. Select a something from the following list that most suits your needs.

*On a fast day eat lightly,*
*enjoy pleasant activities,*
*and rest.*

## One Full Meal Fast

One complete, regular meal may be eaten either at noon or between 6:00 pm and 8:00 pm. Milk, tea, and water may be sipped throughout the day. For non-vegetarians, meat is not eaten during when eating lightly or during a fast.

## A Light Food Fast

Twice a day eat a small amount of light food. Spices, sugar, and salt can be included, if desired. Eat the first meal between 11:30 a.m. and noon, and the second between 6:00 p.m and 7:30 pm.

## Some Foods for a  Light Fast
Unsweetened cereals: cornflakes, puffed rice
puffed wheat, or plain wheat flakes
A steamed small sweet potato or a white potato
A small serving of one of the Light Meal recipes
(See list of recipes)

## A Liquid Fast

Eat no solid food, but three or four times a day during the 24 hours sip a glass of any of the following:

Warm water
Milk—warm or cool
Fruit juice
Coffee or tea
Buttermilk or thin Lassi
Add no salt, sugar, or spices.

## Warm Water Fast

Three or four times a day during a 24-hour period, sip a glass of warm water, but take no solid food.  This is a soothing fast.

## An Annual Fast

It is possible once a year to fast for seven days to maintain health, under a doctor's supervision, and if you want to do it. AyurVeda recommends visiting your physician before undertaking a long fast.  The best time of the year for a seven day fast is in the cloudy, rainy, or cool season of spring or fall when agni is dullest in the environment. Fasting in the extremes of summer or winter is not generally recommended. There are two fasts to choose from. In the first, drink warm water during the daytime only.  In the other kind of fast, water, warm or cool milk, tea, or coffee can be sipped during the day, and small amounts of steamed sweet potatoes, or white potatoes can be eaten at noontime and 6:00 to 7:00 p.m. No salt, sugar, or spices should be added to the food.

An annual fast lasting one week will reduce weight. For those not wanting to gain it back, breaking the fast with careful attention to the amount of food eaten afterward is important. In the weeks following an annual fast eating should continue to be somewhat light. Even after a one-day Complete Fast, a return to eating a lot of heavy foods in pre-fast quantities results in rapid weight gain with greater body weight than before fasting. And this newly acquired weight is particularly difficult to lose.

## Eat Fully

After a weight-reducing fast, eat one-fourth less than usual in both the amount and heaviness of food. By returning to habits of overeating right after an annual fast problems of weight gain and indigestion will be seriously aggravated. If weight gain is not a problem then return to eating normal quantities after fasting. AyurVeda does not recommend extending a fast for more than seven days or long fasting more than once a year.

## Recipes for Light Eating

When following the Light Food Fast , or the One Full Meal fast any of the following recipes from Chapter 10 make a nutritious light meal.

Baked Lentil Soup and Rice

Baked Wild Rice Casserole

Cornbread and Soup or Salad

French Potato Soup (Potage Printanier)

Masoor Dahl and Rice

R & S Couscous

Simple Rice Pilaf

Spinach and Chicory Salad

Tossed Green Saladwith Dressing of Choice

Vegetable Barley Sauté

Vegetables with Roasted and Spiced Barley

Vegetable Soup With Fresh Herbs

## For New Mothers and Their Babies

These dietary recommendations represent only a part of the Maharishi Ayur-Veda Program for Mothers and Babies. For complete information regarding medical consultations and post-delivery treatments in the home contact a Maharishi Ayur-Veda Medical Clinic. We are grateful to the director of the program, Mrs. Clara Berno, in Fairfield, Iowa, for providing this information.

## The New Mother

The first six weeks after giving birth are important for the new mother and her child. AyurVeda calls it *Kaya Kalpa* (KI-ah KUL-puh), a time for rejuvenation, an opportunity to reach perfection. In this six-week program a new mother can reorganize her whole body. The birth process naturally results in fatigue and disturbance of Vata. From that point the Mother and Baby program builds up the entire psycho-physiology to a state of increased balance and strength. The baby benefits greatly from the mother's increased well-being.

*We just give a helping hand to Mother Nature.*
*She set the whole thing up,*
*we just help make it easy.*
- Clara Berno

A new mother is in a physically and emotionally delicate state. After the delivery of a baby, the digestive fire, agni, is often diminished; her digestive system is as delicate as her baby's. The new mother's diet should be specifically designed for her. She neither needs nor can she properly use heavy, sour, or rough foods. Her diet should consist of delicious, warm, nutritious, nourishing, and Vata-balancing recipes. Chicken, fish, and other meats are such heavily concentrated proteins they can not be easily digested. If there is a desire for meat it can be taken as a broth or very thin soup.

# A New Mother's Guidelines for Good Eating

- Eat before nursing
- Never nurse when hungry
- Don't nurse and eat at the same time
- Eat fresh, good quality food
- Eat when you are hungry
- Enjoy your food
- Eat in pleasant surroundings
- Eat sitting down
- Do not eat or cook when you are upset
- Practice moderation in eating
- Follow the body's wisdom for food selection
- Balance the six tastes at every meal
- Eat a suitable amount
- Consider time of day and seasonal changes
- Follow common sense . . . not rigid rules

## Good Digestion

How well a mother's food is digested and assimilated determines the quality of her milk. Following the guidelines for eating well and maintaining a strong digestive fire are necessary for the best assimilation of food. Both good appetizers and beautiful presentation of the meal help to ignite agni. Even something as simple as a tablespoon of warm rice and ghee before eating works. Some new mothers, depending on their physical strength, or strong Pitta nature, will maintain healthy appetites and lively agni right after the birth process. Many others notice that they are not as hungry or able to digest their meals as well as they did before delivery. Whatever the case, it is important to respect the level of digestion the new mother experiences and prepare meals accordingly.

*Appetizers before a meal are like kindling for a fire.*

*To make a roaring blaze,*

*start with paper, sticks, and kindling.*

*Once it's going then throw in a log.*

- Clara Berno

## Balancing Vata

The imbalance in Vata can best be corrected by following a modified Vata-balancing diet, consulting a Maharishi Ayur-Veda physician for special instructions, and by scheduling special in-home treatments. Many mothers enjoy the benefits so much they continue on the new mothers' diet for many months after the six-week program is over. Enjoyment and comfort are the deciding factors.

## Loss of Weight

By carefully following the New Mothers' AyurVeda diet, any weight gained during pregnancy naturally comes off. In fact many mothers say that after childbirth they are able to maintain a more natural weight than they've had in years. This diet also gives her baby a comfortable, healthy start in life.

## Baby's Diet

AyurVeda recommends mother's milk as the best food for a new baby's nourishment and digestion. Breast milk is being developed at the same time the baby is developing. Considering all factors of time, environment, climates, and so forth, mother's milk is specifically good for her own newborn.

## A Mother's Diet and Her Baby

Because of its immature digestive system a newborn baby has an easier time digesting milk if mother follows a Vata-balancing diet. Many of the dietary suggestions in this book for nursing mothers help to nourish their new babies, too. Whatever a mother eats directly affects her baby. By following an Ayur-Vedic diet, she will find that her baby experiences less discomfort of intestinal gas. If a mother is up at night with an uncomfortable, crying baby, the quality of her emotional state as well as increasing fatigue will affect the quality of her milk and the child care she provides.

The most perfect diet for mother and baby is a modified Vata-reducing diet, one that is very simple, wholesome, and easily digested. Items from each food group are simply prepared. Most of the menu is made up of fruit, vegetables, milk, dahl and rice, or other soups.

# The New Mother's Diet

---

## • Warm • Sweet • Oily • Liquid • Soothing •

---

Sweet fruits and vegetables simply steamed until well done are easy to make and comfortable to digest. Stir-fried or sautéed vegetables should be so thoroughly cooked until very soft. Vegetable taste especially good when served in a little seasoned vegetable broth. Eat only *sweet*, thoroughly ripened fruits, such as peaches, pears, mangoes, berries, and cherries.

A new mother should drink at least two cups of warm milk a day with a little ghee added. To warm milk properly, bring it to a boil and then allow it to cool to a comfortable temperature before drinking. A pleasant drink can be made by mixing a cup of warm milk, a teaspoon of ghee, a little sugar, and ground cardamom to taste.

Very soupy dahl and Basmati rice or other long grain rice mixed together make a soothing dish for new mothers. Boil rice in a little extra water to make it plump rather than dry, and add ghee to the water. Mung dahl, from split mung beans, causes less gas than other types. And it is easily digested. Dahl should be well cooked until the beans completely disappear, and be very liquid after cooking. Four or five cups of water for each cup of lentils is a good proportion. Add salt, ghee, and Vata Churna, to taste, while cooking.

## What to Avoid

Of the many foods usually included in a standard Vata-balancing diet a few should be avoided by new mothers. These are: yeast-risen breads and leavened baked goods, cream sauces, chocolate, cheese, tomatoes, such stimulating drinks as coffee, tea, and alcohol, carbonated drinks, sour and heavy foods. Substitute chapatis or heated flour tortillas for leavened bread.

*In the early days a new mother*
*craves a simple diet.*
*After that meals should be*
*sumptuously full of variety.*

- Jan Thatcher, mother of two

# Vata-Balancing Diet for New Mothers

| FAVOR: | Warm, Oily, Sweet, Salty, Liquid Foods |
|---|---|
| Dairy: | Whole milk |
| Sweeteners: | Sugar, Molasses, Honey |
| Oils: | Ghee, Sesame Oil, Olive Oil |
| Grains: | Rice, Wheat (with ghee), Unleavened Baked Goods |
| Fruits: | Sweet Apples, Coconut, Peaches, Cherries, Mango, Papaya, Avocado, Pineapple, Plums, Berries. |
| Vegetables: | Beet, Carrot, Cucumber, Eggplant, Yellow, Butternut and Acorn  Squash, Pumpkin, Spinach |
| Lentils: | Mung Dahl |
| Spices: | Cardamom, Cinnamon, Cumin, Fennel, Fenugreek, Salt, Ginger, Black Pepper (small quantities), Brown Mustard Seeds, Saffron |
| Nuts: | Blanched Almonds, finely ground |
| Animal Foods: | |
| (non-vegetarians) | None in first six weeks.  Broth from chicken or turkey later on, if desired. |

| REDUCE/AVOID: | |
|---|---|
| | Cold, Dry, Very Light or Heavy, Raw Foods, Bitter, Pungent, Astringent Tastes |
| Dairy: | Cheese, Sour Cream, Heavy Cream |
| Grains: | Barley, Oats, Corn, Millet, Buckwheat, Rye |
| Breads: | Leavened with yeast, baking soda, or baking powder |
| Fruits: | Sour Apples and Pears, Pomegranate, Cranberry, Dried Fruit |
| Vegetables: | Peas, Broccoli, Cabbage, Cauliflower, Brussel Sprouts, Potatoes,  Green Leafy and Raw Vegetables |
| Beans: | All Except Mung Lentils |
| Spices: | Allspice, Basil, Cayenne, Coriander, Nutmeg, Turmeric, Oregano, Paprika |
| Animal Food : (non-vegetarians) | All |

201

## Recipes For New Mothers

New mothers in the Maharishi Ayur-Veda Mother and Baby Program often say they prefer eating warm vegetable soups or creamy breakfast cereals. Cream of wheat or rice cereals with a few raisins and finely ground blanched almonds make a nourishing breakfast or supper.  There are many possible variations that can be made from the basic vegetable soup recipe in this section.

These recipes, created by Jan Thatcher and other members of the Mother and Baby Program in Fairfield, Iowa, are tried and tested favorites.  Several of the recipes are baked at the same temperature and can be prepared together to save time.  Sometime in the future, when their babies aren't so new, they hope to write a book with more extensive menu guidelines and recipes, but they offer these as a starting point.

*The baby is the direct recipient of*

*the new mother's increased well-being,*

*health, and happiness.*

-Clara Berno

# Baked Lentil Soup

This extraordinarily neat and easy method of making a delicious dahl is good for everyone, not only new mothers. It's an extremely soupy dahl, best for Vata and Kapha to digest. In a regular diet you might want to double the amount of lentils. New mothers would have only about a quarter of a cup of this soup served over rice.

To save time bake rice in a separate covered casserole in the oven with the soup. Either follow the recipe for Saffron Rice or simply put a cup of rice, 2 1/2 cups of water, 1 tablespoon ghee, and salt (to taste) in baking dish. Cover and bake for half an hour. This can be done at the beginning or end of the Baked Lentil Soup's cooking time.

Serves 3 to 4

    1/3 cup mung lentils, washed and cleaned
    4 cups boiling water
    1/2 teaspoon salt
    1 teaspoon ghee
    1/2 teaspoon Vata Churna
    1/2 cup spinach, chopped (optional)
    1 teaspoon ghee
    1 teaspoon brown mustard seeds
    1 teaspoon Vata Churna

Preheat oven to 350°.

Place ingredients in a 1-quart casserole, cover tightly, and bake for 1 1/2 to 2 hours. It will make a very thin lentil dahl.

To prepare spices:

Heat ghee in a small pan over moderate flame. Add mustard seeds and when they start to pop stir in Churna. Add to cooked dahl, stirring well to combine. Serve with rice.

## Curried Squash Soup

Serves 4 to 6

2 acorn or 1 large butternut squash
2 1/4 cups water or Vata Broth
1/2 teaspoon salt
2 tablespoons ghee
1/2 teaspoon ground cumin
1/2 teaspoon cinnamon
1/4 teaspoon ground cardamom
3/4 teaspoon ground ginger
1 cup orange or apple juice

Preheat oven to 400°.

Split squash lengthwise and bake face-down on an oiled tray for 30 minutes to an hour, or until soft. Cool and scoop out the insides. Makes about 3 cups.

Purée in food processor or blender with the water and salt. Pour into 4-quart pan and heat on low flame. In a small pan heat the ghee and sauté the spices. Add to the soup as it heats. Stir in juice and simmer gently, stirring to blend. When well heated, serve.

## Fresh Spinach Purée

Many recipes in the new mother's diet are appropriate for any convalescents. This is one of them. It is very soothing and easy to digest.

Serves 1

1/2 pound fresh spinach, washed and de-stemmed
1 tablespoon ghee
A pinch of nutmeg
1 teaspoon sesame seeds

Pat spinach with paper towel, place in small saucepan with ghee and nutmeg. Cover and heat over low flame for 7 or 8 minutes or until limp. Stir occasionally to cook evenly. Purée in blender or food processor. Toss in sesame seeds and serve immediately.

## Khichari

This is traditional Indian food for soothing diets. Nutritious and easily digested, Khichari is simply rice and dahl cooked thoroughly together. Total cooking time is about 1 1/2 hours.

Serves 2 to 3

1/4 cup mung lentils, cleaned and washed
1 1/2 cup water
1 teaspoon salt
1 teaspoon Vata Churna
1/4 cup rice
2 tablespoons ghee
1 1/4 cup water
1/4 teaspoon saffron (optional)
1 tablespoon ghee
1 teaspoon cumin
1 teaspoon mustard seeds

Bring water to a boil in a 2-quart pan. Add lentils, salt, and Churna. Cover and bring back to a boil, then reduce heat to very low and simmer for about an hour. Add rice, ghee, water, and saffron. Increase heat and bring to boil again. Then reduce to low and simmer for half an hour. Stir frequently to avoid sticking and add more water if it becomes too thick. Khichari should have the consistency of thick gravy. When ready to serve, heat ghee in small pan with spices. When mustard seeds start to pop stir spices into the soup and serve.

## Quick Vegetable Medley

New mothers find this combination colorful and delicious and very easy to make.

Serves 2

1 tablespoon ghee
1/2 teaspoon ground cumin
1/2 teaspoon Vata Churna
1/2 medium cucumber, peeled, seeded, diced
1 small beet, shredded
1/2 large carrot, shredded

Heat ghee in a skillet over a moderately high flame. Stir in spices and vegetables. Cover and reduce heat to low. Stir frequently, frying until vegetables are well-cooked and soft.

## Simply Baked Carrots

This dish is simple to bake along with Baked Lentil Soup (dahl), but only for half an hour.

Serves 2 to 3

1/2 pound carrots
1/4 cup water
1/4 teaspoon salt
4 tablespoons ghee
1/4 cup sesame seeds

Preheat oven to 350°.

Julienne carrots or cut into narrow finger-length pieces. Place in saucepan with water and salt. Boil over moderately high flame just until tender. test with a fork. Arrange carrots in a small deep baking pan, pour in any remaining liquid along with them. Sprinkle with sesame seeds and ghee. Bake, uncovered, for 30 minutes or until golden brown, and baste several times with juices.

## Sweet Potato-Apple Pie

A little like pumpkin pie this can be served as a sweet main dish for Vata and Pitta diets, or even a dessert. Without the pie crust it's a good side dish that's less heavy to digest.

Makes an 8-inch pie

> 1 unbaked 8-inch pie crust
> 1 large sweet potato, baked
> 1 sweet apple, peeled and shredded
> 1/8 cup sweet orange, pineapple, or apple juice
> 1/4 cup brown sugar
> 1/4 cup blanched almonds, finely ground
>     or
> 1/4 cup coconut
> 1/4 teaspoon cinnamon
> 1/8 teaspoon ginger and nutmeg mixed

Preheat oven to 350°.

Peel potato and mash with other ingredients. Spread mixture onto pie crust. Bake for 30 to 40 minutes or until crust is nicely browned and toothpick inserted in center comes out clean. Cool at least 10 minutes before cutting.

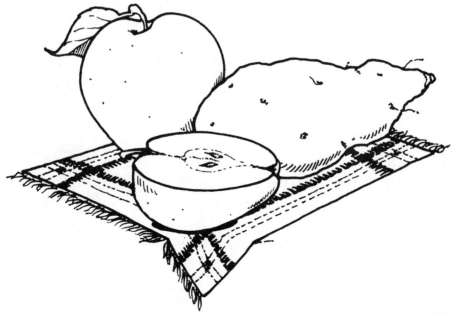

## Sweet Potato Soup

This soup is not only a good one for new mothers but for those with Vata and Pitta constitutions.  If made with cream, omit the salt.

Serves 4 to 6

6 to 7 cups water
4 medium sweet potatoes
2 carrots (use 1 for Pitta)
1 bay leaf
1/2 to 1 cup heavy cream or half and half
              or
   1 cup Vata or Pitta Broth and 1/2 teaspoon salt
2 tablespoons ghee
White pepper, to taste
Cardamom, to taste

Bring water to boil in a large pot.  Meanwhile peel and chop potatoes and carrots.  When water is boiling add bay leaf, salt, and vegetables.  Turn to medium, cover, and cook until soft, or about 40 minutes.  Purée in a food processor or blender until smooth.  Return to pot.  Add enough cream to make a thin soup; add the ghee, and seasonings to taste.  Heat thoroughly and serve.

## Variable Vegetable Soup

This soup is similar to the Vata Broth recipe in Chapter 2, but the vegetables are kept in the soup. Use any combination of Vata-reducing vegetables from the recommended diet.

Serves 4

6 cups water
4 cups mixed vegetables, chopped
1 teaspoon salt, or to taste
1 tablespoon ghee
1 teaspoon brown mustard seeds
1/2 teaspoon cumin, ground
1/2 teaspoon fenugreek, ground
1 teaspoon cardamom, ground
Black pepper, to taste

Bring the water to boil in a large pot. Add vegetables and salt. Cover and simmer for 30 minutes. Heat the ghee in a small frying pan over a medium flame. Add the mustard seeds. When they begin popping add the remaining spices and stir for 30 seconds. Stir into the soup and simmer another hour.

## Lightly Seasoned Vegetables

Vegetables prepared this way make a good side dish or a light evening meal for anyone following a Vata-reducing diet or children who like vegetables.

Serves 4 to 6

1/2 cup carrots, sliced thin
1/2 cup beets, sliced thin
1 cup yellow squash, sliced thin
1/2 cup (or more to taste) spinach,washed and chopped
2 tablespoons ghee
1/2 teaspoon brown mustard seeds
1/2 teaspoon cardamom, ground
1 teaspoon Vata Churna
      or
1/2 teaspoon cumin, ground
8 fenugreek seeds, ground

Cook vegetables in a pressure cooker or steamer until tender.  In a large skillet heat the ghee and mustard seeds.  When the seeds start to pop add the remaining spices and salt.  Stir for 30 seconds and then add the vegetables. Sauté for about 2 minutes or until well coated with the spices.

## Mother's Laddu

These sweet, unctuous (oily) cookies are both nourishing and satisfying. They are good for anyone following a regular Vata-or Pitta-reducing diet. If there is not enough time to roll them into balls, just pat the dough into an 8-inch square pan and allow to set until firm, then cut into 1-inch squares.

Makes about 1 1/2 dozen

>    4 tablespoons ghee
>    3 tablespoons blanched almonds, finely ground
>    1 cup besan (chickpea flour from health food store)
>    6 green cardamom pods, seeded and ground
>             or
>    1/2 teaspoon fresh ground cardamom
>    1 cup brown sugar

In a large skillet or heavy pan heat the ghee. Add ground almonds and besan flour. Cook over low heat stirring frequently until golden. Watch closely so that the flour does not get too dark. Remove from heat and add the other ingredients, stirring well. The dough will leave the sides of the pan and be thick when it is well mixed. Cool just until it can be handled, about 30 minutes. Roll each Laddu into a small ball, smaller than a golf ball. Rub hands with ghee if the dough sticks too much. Arrange them on a plate as they are rolled and set aside for at least an hour, or until they are hard, then serve. Store in a tightly sealed container.

## Simple Shortbread

A rich unleavened dessert for new mothers  It can be served more festively with jam spread on top.

Makes 1 dozen

1/2 pound (2 sticks) butter
1/2 cup sugar—or more to taste
2 cups unbleached flour
1/4 teaspoon salt

Preheat oven to 350°.

Cream butter thoroughly with the sugar.  Mix flour and salt together, then add to the butter mixture.  Roll or pat out dough to 1/4-inch thickness, cut into 1-inch by 2-inch rectangles, prick several times with a fork.  Place with sides not touching on an ungreased baking sheet.  Bake 20 to 25 minutes or until light brown on edges.

Faster Method: Pat dough into a 9-inch pie pan, prick all over the top and bake 25 to 30 minutes.  Cut when warm.

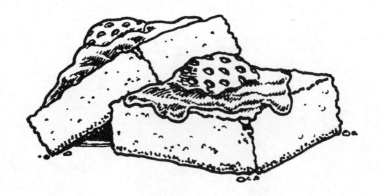

## Other Recipes Good For New Mothers

Some other recipes found in Chapter 10, "An AyurVeda Recipe Companion,"
are good for balancing Vata and appeaing to new mothers.

Puris and Chapatis
Vata Broth
Saffron Rice
( made with extra water)
Couscous
R & S Couscous
Apple Pie and Vanilla Sauce
(or use other sweet fruits in pies and turnovers)
Creamy Rice Pudding
Jam Diagonals

# 9 The AyurVeda Cookbook

*Chapter 10*

# An AyurVeda Recipe Companion

# Contents

Beverages................................................ 215

Appetizers.............................................224

Salads..................................................228

Dressings, Sauces, Dips, Marinades..... 234

Condiments........................................... 241

Other Basics.......................................... 247

Breads.................................................. 252

Soups................................................... 257

Main Dishes...........................................266

Pies and Pastries....................................296

Cookies.................................................307

Cakes...................................................317

Other Desserts.......................................327

## Bed and Breakfast Drink

This is a good beverage to drink in the morning and at bedtime.

1 cup milk per person—low fat for Kapha
1 to 2 teaspoons ghee
Sugar to taste

Heat milk over moderate heat, stirring frequently. When just at boiling point add ghee and sugar. Stir and allow to come to a full boil. Cool and serve warm. For those reducing weight eliminate the ghee and use skim milk.

## Fragrantly Spiced Lassi

This more elaborate Fragrantly Spiced Lassi is served at dinner parties or special occasions. It is served at the end of the meal rather than as an accompanying beverage. If taken in large amounts Lassi increases Pitta and Kapha, otherwise it is good for everyone to drink. Prepare one cup per person if more guest arrive simply add more water.

Makes 1 quart

1 cup plain yogurt
1/2 cup white sugar, or to taste
3 cups cold water
1 green cardamom pod, husked and seeded
    or
1/4 teaspoon ground caramom
Pinch of saffron, crumbled
1/8 teaspoon nutmeg
1 teaspoon rosewater

Mix yogurt and water together in a bowl, beating until smooth. Add water and spices. Stir well, cover, and refrigerate 2 to 4 hours. Just before serving stir in rosewater.

## Indian Spiced Milk Tea

One afternoon when we had talked about food and fasting until we were both too hungry to go on, Dr. Kasture suggested stopping for tea. Even though he claims he is no cook, he made this delicious tea common to his homeland. It is good for anyone who likes to drink black tea and a fine afternoon pick-me-up.

    1 cup milk per serving
    1 tea bag per serving
    1 to 2 teaspoons sugar
    1/8 teaspoon ground cardamom
    1/8 teaspoon cinnamon

Heat milk over moderate heat. When steamy add the other ingredients and stir frequently. Bring just to a boil. Cool before drinking.

**For Kapha:** Use skim or low fat milk and substitute ginger for the cardamom.

## Pineapple Mint Tea

Pineapple is especially useful for balancing Pitta in the summer. This fruity herbal tea is good for everyone to drink, although only those following a Pitta-reducing diet would drink it chilled.

Makes 2 quarts

2 cups fresh mint leaves, washed
or
4 tablespoons dried mint
1 quart boiling water
4 ounces frozen pineapple juice concentrate, defrosted
or
2 cups fresh pineapple juice
3 or 4 sprigs fresh mint for garnish

Put mint in boiling water. Cover right away and remove from heat. Steep for at least 20 minutes. Remove mint and pour tea into pitcher with pineapple concentrate and 1 quart cold water. Stir well. If served as a punch, float a few sprigs of mint on top.

## Plain Refreshing Lassi

Lassi (LAH-see) is good for everyone, especially when served in warm weather and at the end of the meal rather than with food. Buttermilk, having the same digestive purpose, can be diluted with water to any consistency and served in place of lassi.

Makes 1 quart

1 cup plain yogurt
3 cups water

Shake yogurt and water in 1-quart jar or mix well until blended. Serve immediately or very slightly chilled.

## Rose Petal Milkshake

This elegant drink soothes and cools the fires of Pitta in summer. When served warm everyone can drink it year round. Rose petals are said to nourish the heart. When finished sipping the drink use a spoon to eat the remaining petals.

Makes 2 cups

2 cups milk—low fat for Kapha
1 1/2 tablespoons Rose Petal Conserve
1/4 teaspoon vanilla (optional)

Blend or shake thoroughly for one minute. The pieces of rose petals will settle to the bottom of the container. Take care to pour them all out when serving.

## Saffron Milk Tea

This warm and rich drink is excellent for Vata. And, with modifications, it's good for Kapha, too. The saffron is a fine internal "heater," but it increases Pitta. In winter Pitta might enjoy a small amount of this drink.

For each serving:
I cup milk
1 teaspoon ghee
1/2 teaspoon saffron, crumbled
1 teaspoon sugar

Heat milk in a heavy saucepan just to the boiling point. Add remaining ingredients and simmer for about 5 minutes or until the milk is rich yellow color. Cool and serve.

**For Kapha and Weight Watchers:** Use skim milk, omit the ghee, and reduce the sugar to taste.

## Sweet Fruit Smoothies

This is a nourishing, cooling drink for balancing Pitta in the heat of summer. It is sweet, heavy, and cold when made with very ripe sweet fruits.

Mixed fruits such as strawberries, peaches, bananas, kiwis, cherries, blueberries add interest and flavor. Adding sugar helps in the digestion of the milk.

For each 2-cup serving:

    1 cup milk
    1/2 cup ice cream (optional)
    1 cup minced ripe fruit
    1 to 2 teaspoons sugar
    1/4 teaspoon nutmeg or cinnamon (optional)

Whirl all ingredients in a blender or food processor or whisk by hand until blended.

## Three-in-One Samhita Supreme

The combinations of spices, ghee, and milk in this drink make it so nourishing that it might be considered a rasayana. It is good to drink by itself for breakfast and again before bedtime. The first version is good for Vata and Pitta, version two is better for Kapha.

### Version I for Vata and Pitta

For each serving:

> 1 cup warm milk
> 1 teaspoon ghee
> 1 teaspoon sugar, or to taste
> 1/2 teaspoon of spices in this proportion:
>> 3 parts cardamom
>> 1 part cloves
>> 1 part cinnamon

Heat milk and ghee together and bring just to a boil. Stir in sugar and spices. Remove from heat and continue stirring until cool enough to drink.

Make up a small batch of spices ahead of time and use 1/2 teaspoon spice mixture per cup of warm milk.

### Version II for Kapha

For each serving:

> 1 cup warm milk, skim milk best
> 1 teaspoon honey, or to taste
> 1 teaspoon of spices in this proportion:
>> 1 part cardamom
>> 1 part ground ginger
>> 1 part ground cloves
>> 1 part cinnamon

## Watermelon Strawberry Punch

This is a wonderfully refreshing fruit punch for a summer picnic or for cooling off on a hot afternoon. Watermelon is good for everyone to eat in the summer. Many other fresh fruit combinations are great with watermelon juice, too. Add small amounts of bottled juices, if you like, but there is so much fresh fruit available in the summer it is easy to make delicious fresh drinks.

The most attractive bowl for this punch is the hollowed watermelon itself although any large bowl will do. Garnish with fresh herbs and flowers, but be sure to use washed flowers or leaves that you *know* are edible.

Makes about 3 quarts

    1 round watermelon, about 12 to 15 pounds
    1 pint strawberries, washed and drained
    2 tablespoons sugar (optional)
    2 limes, thinly sliced
    Sprigs of fresh mint and lemon balm
    Blossoms from borage (blue shooting stars), nasturtium, pineapple sage, sweet violets, etc.

To Prepare Watermelon Punchbowl:

Wash and dry melon. Cut 1/4-inch slice off the bottom so it will stand upright. Mark the melon about one third from the top and slice open. This small top piece can be saved for use as a cover. To save the juices work on a cookie sheet with sides or a large shallow pan. Remove as much melon as you can in large chunks, then scrape the inside clean. Use a melon baller to make about 2 cups of balls, or cut into bite-size cubes and reserve. Be sure to remove all seeds. Juice the remaining watermelon by pounding it in a deep bowl and then straining through a sieve or use a food mill. You will have about 2 to 2 1/2 quarts of melon juice.

Pour juice into melon shell or serving bowl. Mix in sugar, if needed.

Juice strawberries in a food mill or strainer and stir into the punch bowl. Add a few ice cubes or serve them in a separate bowl. Garnish with melon balls, lime slices, mint leaves, and flowers.

## Cheese Crackers

These appetizers are more like soft little biscuits than crackers. Traditionally they are served warm with a selection of Italian cheeses, such as Parmesan, fontini, and mozzarella. Pitta should eat lightly from the cheese tray. Whether eaten by themselves or with soup, these little cheese crackers add a salty taste that is slightly pungent and sweet. Eating them reduces Vata, is neutral for Pitta, and increases Kapha.

Serves 6 generously

1 cup flour
1/2 teaspoon salt
1/2 teaspoon paprika
Coarsely ground black pepper to taste
1/2 cup butter
1 cup grated cheese—Parmesan, Romano, or cheddar in combination
2 tablespoons heavy cream
1/2 tablespoon heavy cream for glaze

Preheat oven to 325°.

Stir the flour together with the salt, paprika, and pepper. With a pastry cutter or the steel knife of a food processor, cut the butter in until it is mealy. Stir in heavy cream. When you have a smooth dough, chill it for about an hour.

Roll out the dough on a floured surface to a thickness of about 1/4 inch. Cut into strips 1/2 inch by 1 1/2 inches. Brush with the cream and arrange on ungreased baking sheets. Bake for 12 to 14 minutes until puffy and a little brown.

## Curried Herb Cheese Dip

Serve this sour, pungent little dip with crackers, chips, or raw vegetables.

Makes 1 cup

- 1/2 cup sour cream
- 1/2 cup ricotta cheese
- 1 tablespoon lemon juice
- 3 tablespoons parsley, minced
- 1 tablespoon basil, minced
- 1/2 teaspoon dry mustard
- 1/2 teaspoon paprika
- 1/4 teaspoon ground white pepper
- A pinch cayenne pepper
- 1/2 teaspoon cumin seeds

In a small bowl cream sour cream and cheese thoroughly. Mix in lemon juice, parsley, basil, mustard, paprika, and peppers. Roast cumin seeds in a hot iron pan until just turning light brown, then grind finely and add to mixture. Spoon into serving bowl, cover, and chill in refrigerator for 2 or 3 hours to set the flavors.

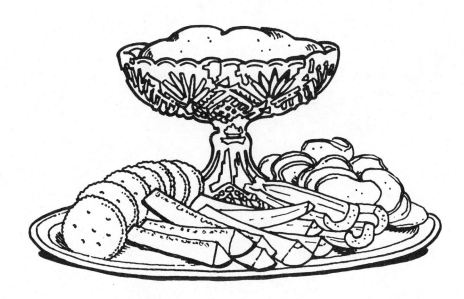

## Fresh Ginger Lemon Chutney

A good appetizer for Vata and Kapha, this chutney is a pleasant accompaniment to many meals besides Indian ones. Left over, this chutney is especially delicious fried with vegetables, or tossed with hot rice or other cooked grains.

Makes 1/2 cup

1 lemon
1/4 pound fresh ginger, peeled
1/2 teaspoon salt
1/2 teaspoon sugar, optional

Peel the lemon with a vegetable peeler or zester. Then mince or chop the peel very fine. Squeeze lemon juice into a small cup. Chop ginger into small chunks in a blender or food processor for 30 seconds. Measure 1/2 cup ginger and leave it in the blender container. Add lemon peel, 1/2 teaspoon lemon juice, salt, and sugar. Blend again for 30 seconds or until the mixture looks soft and tan. Serve in a tiny bowl or dish. It keeps one day.

# Golden Yummies

These delicious little appetizers are sweet, oily, and a little pungent. They are good for all doshas when served as hot hors d'oeuvres. Allow 2 to 3 per person. The topping is good by itself as a sweet condiment or chutney.

Makes 2 cups

For the Topping:

    1 1/2 tablespoons ghee
    1/2 teaspoon cayenne
    1/3 cup milk or cream
    1 to 2 tablespoons sugar, to taste
    1/8 teaspoon allspice
    1/8 to 1/4 teaspoon saffron, crushed
    1/4 cup raisins
    1 to 1 1/2 cups coconut—finely chopped is best, but flaked will do

In a small saucepan or frying pan, heat ghee over moderately high flame. Then add cayenne and stir about 1 minute. Add milk, sugar, allspice, and crumbled saffron threads. Bring to a boil, stirring often. Milk should begin turning golden yellow. Reduce heat to simmer. Stir in raisins and 1 cup coconut. Beat well as the mixture leaves sides of the pan. If it is too liquid, add more coconut a tablespoon at a time until the mixture is just moist but not wet. Set aside until ready to assemble, or serve as a chutney.

To Assemble:

    1/2 tablespoon ghee
    1/8 teaspoon cayenne
    Cashew, almond, or sesame nut butter
    Wheat or other mild flavored crackers

Heat the ghee and cayenne in a small pan. Add 2 or 3 tablespoons of topping per person. Fry over high heat, stirring until heated thoroughly. Spread each cracker with 1/2 teaspoon nut butter, then top with 1 teaspoon hot coconut mixture. Serve warm.

If prepared in advance, put under broiler for 30 seconds before serving.

A Vata/Kapha suggestion: To make a big Golden Yummie that is a satisfying part of a light meal. Use a large rice cake or a slice of toast instead of crackers.

## Pineapple Ginger-Cream Spread

This sweet, pungent, and sour little sandwich spread is best for Vata butboth Pitta and Kapha can enjoy some spread on a cracker or two. It makes a fine celery stuffing for a party relish tray.

Makes 1 cup

    8 ounces cream cheese
    1/4 cup fresh ginger, chopped
    2 1/2 tablespoons crushed pineapple, drained
    1/2 teaspoon nutmeg
    1/4 teaspoon cardamom, ground

Mix all ingredients together thoroughly. Cover and set aside in refrigerator an hour before serving.

## Asparagus Salad in Raspberry Vinaigrette

A colorful and unusual salad. that is good for Vata, neutral for Pitta, and increases Kapha slightly. It adds sweet, a little sour, and astringent tastes to the meal.

Serves 4

> 10 asparagus stalks
> Lettuce leaves
> Raspberry vinaigrette--see below
> Coarsely ground pepper
> 1/2 teaspoon salt

Clean asparagus and steam whole stalks. When tender, yet a bright green, immediately blanch in cold water to retain the color. Refrigerate until just cool.

When ready to serve arrange the spears on lettuce leaves. Pour raspberry vinaigrette dressing over the middle of the spears. Sprinkle with salt and coarsely ground pepper.

## Raspberry Vinaigrette

> 2 tablespoons white vinegar
> 1/2 cup light oil, safflower or sunflower
> 1/4 teaspoon salt
> 1 cup of fresh raspberries, washed,
> > or
> 10 ounces frozen raspberries, defrosted

Mix vinegar, salt, and oil in a jar with tight fitting lid. Put raspberries in a sieve to drain. Purée by mashing against the sides with a wooden spoon. Mix raspberry purée with an equal part of the vinaigrette dressing. Shake very well before serving.

229

## Coleslaw With Caraway Dressing

This salad adds the sour taste to Pitta's diet and should be served as part of a balanced meal that includes other Pitta-reducing dishes, rather than being eaten by itself. Although the sour tastes of caraway, sour cream, and yogurt in the dressing are good additions to Vata's diet, the cabbage makes this salad a side dish to be eaten in moderation by Vata. The dressing could be used on other green salads or it can be heated and served over steamed cabbage. Kapha would infrequently eat coleslaw.

Makes 4 to 6 servings

    1 teaspoon caraway seeds
    1/4 cup sour cream
    1/8 cup plain yogurt
    1 teaspoon sugar
    1/2 teaspoon vinegar
    1/2 medium head cabbage, finely shredded

In a small heavy pan toast the caraway seeds over a low flame. Stir constantly until light brown. Remove from heat and crush with mortar and pestle or in spice grinder. Whisk sour cream, yogurt, and sugar in a small bowl. Add the caraway and vinegar. Then toss thoroughly with the shredded cabbage. Cover and chill for at least an hour before serving.

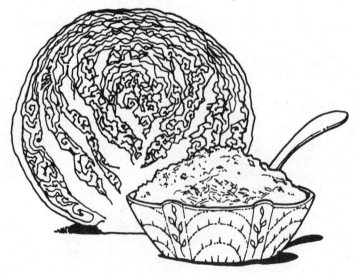

## Confetti Rice Salad

This is a pleasant summertime party salad this is especially good for Vata and Pitta. Kapha can eat this rice dish in moderation with a green leafy salad or separately as a light meal. This is a light, sweet, cold dish with some bitter, pungent, and sour tastes.

Makes 4 cups

> 2 1/2 cups cooked rice
> 1/2 yellow pepper, chopped
> 1/2 sweet red pepper chopped
> 1 full stalk celery (with leaves), chopped
> 4 tablespoons fresh parsley, chopped
> 1 1/2 tablespoons mixed fresh herbs of choice, such as basil, tarragon,
> summer savory, fennel, finely minced
> 5 tablespoons vinaigrette dressing
> Salt and pepper to taste
> Chopped parsley and paprika, optional garnish

While rice is still warm, toss with chopped vegetables, herbs, and dressing. Add salt and pepper to taste. Sprinkle on extra chopped parsley, or a little sweet paprika for color. Cover and chill for 2 or 3 hours. Serve on a bed of lettuce with wedges of tomato and sliced cucumber.

Suggestion: Sauté leftover rice salad in oil with vegetables for a satisfying side dish or light meal.

## Simple Vinaigrette Dressing

> 1/4 cup oil
> 1 tablespoon warm water
> 1 tablespoon vinegar
> 1/4 teaspoon salt

Place all ingredients in a small jar, cover tightly, and shake vigorously.

## Macedonia di Fruita

All the fruits in this salad are good for the all doshas when eaten as a part of a meal, but it would not be good for Kapha as a separate meal.  The white Calmyrna figs are known by the name *anjier* and are considered one of the greatest of all fruits.  This is an excellent salad or dessert to serve Pitta in the summer.

For the culinary artist these fruits are like colors on a palette waiting to be made into something spectacular.  When prepared in a grand manner this dish can be used as an impressive centerpiece for a buffet dessert.

Serves 8 to 10

>    4 apples, sweet, not tart
>    3 sweet oranges
>    1 large cantaloupe, balls or cubes
>    2 cups cubed watermelon
>    1 medium honeydew melon, balls or cubes
>            or
>    Any other melon varieties in season
>    8 to 12 Calmyrna figs
>    8 to 10 small bunches unsprayed grapes, red, green, and deep purple
>    10 to 12  pitted dates
>    Other seasonal fruits of choice

Core and thickly slice the apples.  Wash the oranges thoroughly and slice with their skins on, or peel and section.  Cube or ball the melons.  Clip the washed grapes into individual bunches.  Arrange the fruits in little groups of 8 to 10 with some of every fruit in each group.  Individual servings can be made ahead of time.

## Spinach and Chicory Salad

The bitter, astringent, slightly pungent, light, hot, and dry properties of this salad are especially balancing for a Kapha diet. It is also a good salad to prepare when serving people with varied dietary needs. If the meal consists of several heavy or sweet dishes, then those following a Kapha diet can help themselves to a large amount of this healthy salad. Vata and Pitta types would eat smaller portions.

Serves 4

1/4 cup basic vinaigrette dressing
1 teaspoon dry mustard
2 teaspoons Kapha Churna
          or
  1 teaspoon coarsely ground black pepper
  1/2 teaspoon ground fenugreek
  1/4 teaspoon ground cumin
  1/4 teaspoon ground coriander
2 cups spinach, washed and torn into bite-size pieces
1 small head chicory—radicchio type
1/2 cup red cabbage, thinly shredded
3 to 4 red radishes, thinly sliced
3 tablespoons blanched, slivered almonds optional

Mix vinaigrette, mustard, and Kapha Churna together. If a spice blend is used instead of the Churna, then mix the dry spices together before adding to the vinaigrette.

Place spinach in a serving bowl and pour vinaigrette over it. Toss well. Add remaining vegetables. Toss again, cover, and refrigerate for at least 30 minutes. Before serving sprinkle with almonds.

## Splendid Layers Salad

A layered, rather "thick" salad that is good at a picnic or served as a light meal on a summer evening. The tastes are sweet, bitter, astringent, and slightly salty. It has oily, cold, and heavy qualities. This combination is good for Pitta types since the heavier vegetables provide enough substance for Pitta's healthy appetite. When eaten in small amounts this salad is all right for Vata, but the cold and heavy qualities aggravate Kapha Be sure to cut everything into bite-size pieces when preparing. Each vegetable can be cut in a different shape to add visual interest.

Serves 6 to 8

> 2 heads of bibb lettuce
> 1/2 head red cabbage, shredded
> 6 large artichoke hearts, steamed and quartered
> > or
> Prepared artichokes: 14-ounce can, drained and quartered or
> > 10 ounces frozen, defrosted and quartered
> 1 pound asparagus, cut in 1-inch pieces and steamed
> 1 cucumber, washed, scored with tines of fork, sliced very thin
> 1 medium jicama or 3 sunchokes, cut in triangular shapes and sliced
> 4 tablespoons Pitta Churna Salad Dressing (recipe follows)
> 4 large leaves Romaine lettuce, de-ribbed, cut in 1 inch squares
> 1 tablespoon fresh mint, dill, and/or fennel
> 1/3 cup curly parsley leaves, broken in clusters
> 1/4 cup small seedless grapes or raisins
> 1 cup mixed salad greens, as available, such as arugula, beet leaves, hon
> > tsai tai, chicory, escarole torn or chopped in small pieces
> 1 red apple, cored and diced
> 1/4 cup croutons, toasted

To Assemble:

Line the bottom and sides of a deep, straight-sided glass bowl or saladbowl with Bibb lettuce leaves. Sprinkle with enough red cabbage to cover the bottom. Layer with about one third of the "thick" ingredients: artichoke hearts, asparagus, cucumber, and jicama. Pour one tablespoon Pitta Churna Dressing over this layer. Begin next layer with a sprinkling of red cabbage and Romaine pieces about an inch thick.

## Splendid Layers Salad, continued

Spread on half of the chopped fresh herbs. Arrange another third of the "thick" ingredients and add the grapes or raisins. Sprinkle with a little red cabbage for color and pour on one tablespoon Pitta Churna dressing to end this layer. Then cover the surface with mixed chopped greens. Sprinkle with the remaining cabbage, herbs, the last third of the vegetables, diced apple, and remaining salad dressing in that order. Ring the outside with parsley clusters and sprinkle croutons in the center. Be sure the bibb lettuce lines the edges of the bowl attractively. Add more leaves, if necessary, to fill in empty spaces. Cover and refrigerate one or two hours before serving.

## Pitta Churna Dressing

Pitta Churna, an AyurVedic blend of herbs and spices especially good for those following a Pitta diet, is useful in soups, dressings, and vegetable and fruit dishes.

    1/2 cup oil, sunflower or safflower
    2 tablespoons warm water
    1 1/2 to 2 teaspoons Pitta Churna
    1/2 teaspoon salt
    2 tablespoons vinegar

Place all ingredients in a jar or blender. Cover tightly and blend well. Let mixture stand for 5 to 10 minutes and blend again. Shake well before serving.

## Tossed Green Salad

An American standard, the tossed green salad is good for everyone in one or another of its many forms. In planning balanced menus a green salad helps in contributing some of the bitter, astringent, and pungent tastes we sometimes have difficulty adding in our main dishes. An interesting tossed green salad made up of several types of lettuce and other fresh greens adds texture and color to a meal. With touches of such fresh herbs as chopped French tarragon, basil (especially tasty cinnamon, anise, and lemon basil leaves) lemon balm, mints, chopped parsley, or cilantro, you'll enjoy many pleasant little surprises as you eat.

Greens should be torn into bite-size pieces. You shouldn't be forced to chop through a tossed salad with a knife, or have to eat large lettuce leaves whole. If the salad is to be a main part of the meal, allow about 1 loosely packed quart of greens for every 2 people. Use fewer greens if many dishes are to be served. It is best to dress a salad just before it is eaten. Any greens that have been dressed with oil should not be saved.

Tossed green salads are especially good for Pitta and Kapha. Keep Kapha's salads light by using just a variety of mixed greens, herbs, and sprouts. By adding such vegetables as tomatoes, avocado, and cucumbers you create a Vata salad.

## Dressings, Sauces, Marinades, and Dips

A good simple salad dressing is a squeeze of lemon juice or a little oil and vinegar. The following salad dressings are good for all body types when mixed well and combined with a green salad. Add various fruits and vege- tables as seasonally availbale to the salad depending on the needs of each body type. Some of the dressings serve also as excellent marinades or sauces to be poured over hot, steamed vegetables.

A flavorful herbal vinegar makes a unique starting point for many vinai- grettes. If you grow some of your own herbs, or know someone who has a lot to spare, making fancy herbal vinegars and oils is easy and well worth the time.

## To Make Basic Herbal Vinegar

1 gallon undiluted, first quality white vinegar—Heinz is best
(other flavored vinegars compete with the subtle herbs)
3 to 4 cups de-stemmed fresh herbs

Pour out about 2 cups of vinegar and save. Wash the herbs, pat dry, and push into the gallon bottle. Top off with reserved vinegar and cap. Turn over gently a few times to saturate everything. Label and date the bottle, if you are making more than one gallon. Set aside in a dark place for 2 or 3 months or up to a year. It is not necessary or even recommended to heat the vinegar before using. There's too great a chance of "cooking" the herbs, thus changing their essential flavors. The astringency of the vinegar naturally draws the flavor out of the plant. For stronger vinegar or when using especially delicate herbs or flowers, remove the leaves after a month and repeat the process with new fresh material.

## To Make Flavored Cooking/Salad Oil

Use fresh mints, thyme, anise, marjoram, rose petals, chive blossoms, and other flavorful, edible herbs in combinations or alone.

1 to 2 cups leaves or flower petals
3 cups  unflavored, cold pressed oil: safflower, sunflower, etc.

Wash herbs, pat dry, and put in a 1-quart jar. Pour oil nearly to the top. Gently shake 2 or 3 times.

The plant's oils are extracted and concentrated in the oil. Gentle heat is needed, but it is not necessary to heat the oil. Just set the bottle in the sun or on a sunny windowsill for 4 or 5 days, gently shaking each day.  Strain and repeat with fresh material at least 2 or 3 times until the scent is distinctly noticeable.

Using good quality green olive oil for basils, oregano, fennel, and herbs results in a delicious oil for Italian cuisine.  You can also add whole allspice or cloves.

## Herbed Vinaigrette

Use plain oil and vinegar or try different combinations of your own flavored oils and vinegars for greater variety.

2 tablespoons herbal vinegar
1/2 teaspoon salt
1/2 cup olive oil
2 tablespoons warm water
1 teaspoon chopped fresh herbs such as parsley, tarragon, thyme, salad burnet or if fresh herbs are not available, use 1/2 teaspoon crushed dry herbs

Place all ingredients in a jar, cover tightly and shake well.  Let mixture stand for a few minutes, then shake well again before serving.

## Avocado Cheese Sauce and Dip

A warm, rich dressing for baked potatoes and other vegetables this sauce is good to serve warm as a vegetable crudité dip. It can be part of a light evening meal, or as a side dish sauce anytime for Vata and Pitta. It is sweet, slightly sour, a little pungent, heavy, and oily. A dramatic way to serve this poured over a whole steamed head of caulifower centered on a large plate and ringed with a variety of small steamed vegetables.

Makes 2 cups.

1 medium ripe avocado
1 teaspoon lemon juice
1 teaspoon sweet paprika
1 cup ricotta or soft panir cheese
1 tablespoon minced fresh herbs: dill, chervil, cilantro, tarragon,
    fennel, parsley, marjoram,
1 teaspoon coarsely ground pepper
1/2 to 3/4 cup heavy cream
1/2 cup milk

Peel avocado and mash with lemon juice and paprika in a bowl or food processor. Add the cheese, herbs, and pepper. Blend until very smooth. Bring the cream and milk to a boil in a 2-quart saucepan. Reduce to simmer and stir in cheese mixture. Stir until well-blended. If sauce seems too thick, add more cream until it pours like thick gravy. Serve warm.

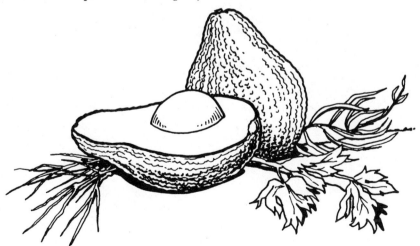

## Basic Cheese Sauce

An all-purpose, sweet, heavy, oily sauce that can be served on steamed vegetables and baked potatoes, this not-very-sour cheese sauce is best for Vata and Pitta. Macaroni and Cheese made with this sauce is more Pitta-balancing than that made with hard, sour cheese. Mixed vegetable casseroles baked with cheese sauce can be served as a side dish for everyone at a main meal. Vary the flavors by adding the spice combination or Churna  you like best.

Makes 2 cups

2 tablespoons ghee or butter
2 tablespoons flour
1 tablespoon Churna or mixed spices of choice
1/2 teaspoon turmeric
3/4 teaspoon finely ground pepper
1 cup heavy cream
1 cup ricotta cheese, mashed

Heat ghee in a heavy pan over low heat.  Add flour and stir to blend.  Add spices and continue stirring until well mixed and thickened.  Slowly whisk in cream and stir vigorously to avoid lumps.  Turn to moderate heat and add the cheese.  Cook uncovered, stirring frequently until sauce is thick and creamy. Serve warm.

# Dressings, Sauces, Dips, Marinades

## Cream Tahini Sauce

This is an easy to make, all purpose sauce to dress up steamed vegetables, baked potatoes, and mixed casseroles. Although it is best for Vata types, Pitta and Kapha can have moderate amounts as part of a balanced meal. This sauce adds sweet, astringent, bitter, oily, hot, and heavy aspects to a meal.

Makes 1 1/2 cups

  1 cup heavy cream
  1/2 cup (8 tablespoons) sesame tahini-- available at natural food stores)
  1/2 teaspoon ground ginger (increase to 1 teaspoon for Kapha)
  1/4 teaspoon ground cloves (optional)
  1/8 teaspoon black pepper

Heat cream in a small pan over moderate heat. When fully boiling turn heat to low and add tahini and spices. Stir until well blended. Serve warm.

## Deanna's Vinaigrette

  5 tablespoons olive oil or other salad oil
  Juice of 1/2 a lime (about 1 tablespoon)
  1 teaspoon prepared mustard—stoneground or Dijon are good
  1 teaspoon honey
  Salt and pepper to taste

Place all ingredients in a covered jar and shake well .

## Ginger Soy Gravy

This delicious, nourishing gravy comes from Bruce Rash, chef at the exclusive Maharishi Ayur-Veda Health Center in Lancaster, Massachusetts. When served as part of a balanced meal it is good for everyone.  It adds salty, pungent, oily, and hot aspects to the meal. This dark, moderately thick gravy is especially good served with mashed potatoes because the ginger helps both Vata and Kapha in digesting heavy potatoes.

Makes 4 cups

> 1/2 cup ghee or cooking oil
> 1/4 cup flour
> 1 tablespoon ground ginger
>           or
>    1/4 cup freshly grated ginger
> 4 cups unflavored soy milk, available at many supermarkets and health food stores.
> 1/4 soy sauce or tamari

In 2-quart saucepan heat oil over moderate heat.  Add flour and stir constantly for about 5 minutes until blended and flour turns light brown. Add ginger and heat another 5 minutes, stirring frequently. Meanwhile, bring the soy milk just to a boil in a separate pan.  Add it slowly to the oil mixture, stirring vigorously with a whip to avoid lumps.  Stir in soy sauce.  Simmer until thick stirring frequently.

## Pitta Churna Salad Dressing and Marinade

Pitta Churna, that special blend of spices and herbs especially good for balancing Pitta dosha, does not need to be heated, as some spices do, to bring out its subtle flavors. This dressing adds a unique flavor to tossed summer salads. It is a pleasant marinade for tofu, eggplant, and other ingredients in a main dish. Both Vata and Kapha can enjoy this dressing, or substitute the appropriate churna as you prefer.

1/2 cup oil, sunflower or safflower
2 tablespoons warm water
1 1/2 to 2 teaspoons Pitta Churna
1/2 teaspoon salt
2 tablespoons vinegar

Place all ingredients in a jar or blender. Cover tightly and blend well. Let mixture stand for 5 to 10 minutes and blend again. Shake well before serving.

## Scrumptious Sesame-Orange Dressing and Sauce

This recipe is also great as a vegetable and cracker dip, a condiment to be served in a small bowl with Indian food, and as a sauce for steamed vegetables.

1/2 teaspoon cumin seeds
5 tablespoons sesame tahini (from specialty groceries or natural food
    stores)
Juice of 1 medium to large orange
Salt and pepper to taste

Toast cumin seeds in a heavy skillet until just brown. Crush with mortar and pestal or in a spice grinder. Mix all ingredients thoroughly.

243

## Apple-Raisin Chutney

Chutneys are good in moderation for balancing all doshas when they are served as part of a meal. This recipe is especially nourishing for Vata dosha. The addition of Kapha Churna gives a pungent taste making it better for Kapha types. It is sweet, pungent, hot, and a little astringent, and it helps maintain the appetite when eaten throughout the meal.

Apple-Raisin Chutney can be saved in capped, sterilized jars in the refrigerator for a month. By substituting Pitta Churna for the Kapha Churna and reducing it to 1 teaspoon, or to taste, this recipe makes a tasty turnover filling for a Vata and Pitta dessert.

Makes 2 1/2 cups

2 cups apples, peeled and chopped
1/2 cup water
1 teaspoon nutmeg
1/4 teaspoon cloves
3 to 4 tablespoons white sugar
1/4 cup brown sugar
2 tablespoons Kapha Churna
1 cup raisins

Put the apples in a large pan. Add the other ingredients and cook over moderate heat, adding more water 1/4 cup at a time to keep chutney from drying out. Stir frequently until apples are tender and transparent, about 30 minutes. Stir well to blend into a sauce. Cool and serve. Store in refrigerator.

## Coconut Chutney

When served as an appetizer or condiment with the meal this rich, golden chutney adds sweet, pungent, oily, heavy properties to the meal.

Makes about 1 1/2 cups

    1 tablespoon ghee
    3/4 teaspoon cayenne
    1/4 cup milk or cream
    1 to 2 tablespoons sugar, to taste
    1/8 teaspoon allspice
    1/8 to 1/4 teaspoon saffron, crushed
    1/4 cup raisins
    1 cup dried coconut (finely chopped is best, but flaked will do)

Heat ghee over medium flame in a small pan. Then add cayenne and stir about one minute. Stir in milk, sugar, allspice, and crumbled saffron threads. Bring to a boil, stirring often. Milk should begin turning golden yellow. Reduce to simmer. Stir in raisins and coconut. Beat well as mixture leaves sides of the pan. If it is too liquid, add more coconut, a tablespoon at a time, until the mixture is just moist but not wet. Serve in a small bowl.

## Fresh Green Chutney

This is a fresh or "daily" chutney that should not be kept as a leftover into the next day. It is astringent, bitter, pungent, a little sweet, and salty. A little eaten with a meal is good for all everyone's digestion and refreshes the palate.

Makes 1 cup

1 cup chopped fresh parsley, coriander leaves, and/or spinach

    1 teaspoon salt
    1 lemon or lime, juiced
    1 teaspoon cayenne, or less, to taste
    1/4 cup water
    1/4 cup dried coconut

Put all ingredients in a blender or food processor with a steel blade. Blend on low speed. Put in serving dish and set aside for 1 to 2 hours before serving.

245

## Kashmiri Mint Chutney

As with other chutneys, mint chutney is good for all doshas as part of a balanced meal, especially for Kapha and Pitta. The tastes in this chutney are astringent, sour, pungent, slightly sweet, and bitter. This chutney keeps only for 1 day.

Makes 1 cup

2/3 cup fresh mint leaves, washed, dried, minced
1/4 cup ground walnuts
1 teaspoon yogurt
1/2 teaspoon turmeric

Mix minced mint leaves and walnuts together. In a small cup stir yogurt and turmeric together, then blend with mint. Cover and allow to sit for 30 minutes before serving.

## Quick Condiments

Here are a few easy condiments that add taste, texture, color and more variety to an Indian dinner. Small bowls and dishes of chutneys and condiments make the meal both interesting to the eye and the palate.

## Lemon and Lime Wedges

Wedged lemons and limes are good to serve at any main meal. They add both color and a sour taste, help clear the palate when eaten with the heavier parts of the dinner, and in small quantities, they aid digestion. Cut washed lemons and limes in narrow wedges and arrange in alternating colors on a small plate.

## Spiced Cashew Nuts

A few of these sweet, oily, slightly heavy nuts are good for Vata and Pitta, and increase Kapha, especially if they are eaten in excess (easy to do). They keep well on the kitchen shelf or in the refrigerator.

Makes 1 cup

1 1/2 tablespoons ghee
1 cup unsalted cashew nuts, broken in pieces
1/2 teaspoon of *one* of the following ground spices:
cardamom, ginger, nutmeg, cinnamon, or coriander

Heat ghee in a small pan over moderate heat. Sprinkle in nuts and spice. Stir frequently until nuts are toasty brown. Serve in a small bowl. If saved for another meal, reheat briefly over a low flame.

## Toasted Coconut Condiment

Serve a small dish of coconut plain or toasted so it can be sprinkled over some favorite curry on the dinner plate. If toasted coconut is served as a condiment, do not serve coconut chutney as well. A little of the sweet, heavy and oily properties of coconut go a long way. They are good for Vata and Pitta, and increase Kapha.

1 tablespoon ghee
1/2 to 2/3 cup flaked coconut
1/4 teaspoon saffron, crumbled (optional)

Heat ghee in a small pan over low heat. Toss in coconut and saffron, stir frequently until it is just brown on the tips. Put in serving dish immediately.

## Tomato Chutney

Everyone can eat some of this chutney as part of a balanced meal, but it increases Pitta dosha if eaten in any more than a small quantity. It has sour, pungent, astringent, sweet, salty, oily, and slightly bitter properties. This cooked chutney keeps well for two weeks tightly covered in the refrigerator.

Makes 2 cups

To Prepare Spices:

> 1 tablespoon ghee
> 1 teaspoon brown mustard seeds
> 1/2 teaspoon fenugreek, ground
> 1 teaspoon cumin seeds, dry roasted and ground
> 1 teaspoon coriander, ground
> 1 teaspoon freshly grated ginger
> > or
> 3/4 teaspoon ground ginger
> 1/2 teaspoon turmeric

Heat ghee in a heavy pot over moderate heat. Add mustard seeds and when they start to pop stir in the other spices. Fry for one minute, stirring constantly.

For the Tomato Mixture:

> 10 medium tomatoes, peeled and mashed
> 1 teaspoon salt
> 1/4 teaspoon sweet paprika (optional)
> 1 tablespoon brown sugar, or to taste
> 1 teaspoon lemon juice

Add the tomatoes to the spices, then stir in the remaining ingredients. Turn to simmer and heat for 10 to 15 minutes, stirring until everything is thoroughly blended. Cover and allow to cook on low for another 10 minutes. Cool and serve.

## Raita

1 to 2 cups plain yogurt
1/4 teaspoon cumin, freshly roasted and ground


Stir yogurt into a serving bowl. Sprinkle most of the cumin on top and stir in. Sprinkle the rest on top. Cover and refrigerate 30 minutes before serving.


## Tomato and Cucumber Raita

A refreshing raita that adds sour and slightly salty tastes to the meal, and cold, heavy qualities.

Makes 2 cups


1 small cucumber, peeled, seeded, and chopped
1/2 teaspoon salt
2 cups plain yogurt
1 medium tomato, skinned and chopped
1/2 teaspoon cumin seeds, roasted and ground


Mix cucumber and salt together in a small glass or stainless steel bowl. Set aside for about 15 minutes to drain the liquid out of the cucumber. Mix yogurt and tomato together in a serving bowl. Squeeze the juice from the cucumber until it feels dry and add it to the yogurt. Discard the juice. Stir in 1/4 teaspoon cumin. Sprinkle the rest on top. Cover tightly and refrigerate 30 minutes to an hour before serving.

## Panir and Ricotta Soft Cheese

This is a good, easily digestible cheese for Vata to eat regularly and the only cheese Pitta should use because it is not as sour as hard cheeses. It is slightly sour, oily, and cold. It can be used in fillings for manicotti and pasta shells, or fried in ghee until crisp then tossed with spiced vegetables.

Makes 1 1/2 cups

2 quarts of milk
2 tablespoons lemon juice or white vinegar
1/2 cup yogurt (optional)

In a heavy pot bring milk to boil over moderately high heat. Watch it carefully so it doesn't boil over. As foam begins rising, remove from heat and stir in juice or vinegar, and the yogurt, if it is used. Continue stirring gently as curds separate from whey. Set aside for five minutes and line a large sieve or colander with enough muslin cheesecloth or a clean, loosely woven towel to tie into a bag.

Pour the cheese into the lined sieve, reserving the whey separately in lidded jars. Drain until cool. Then wrap the cloth tightly around the curds and squeeze out excess liquid. Hang the bag over a bowl or above the sink for an hour until most of the liquid is gone. Then press the cheese, slightly kneading it for panir, into a shallow pan or sealable container. Cover and refrigerate for 5 or 6 hours or overnight. Ricotta usually contains more liquid and is hung for less time, if at all. It does not have be kneaded and refrigerated, but can be used right away.

# To Make Ghee

In a heavy saucepan melt a pound or more of butter over medium heat. When butter becomes liquid and foamy turn the heat to low. Simmer slowly for about an hour skimming the froth off every once in a while. Unless the ghee is made from fresh, unsalted butter (not the commercial variety) discard the skimmings. Otherwise these are a nutritious addition to rice, bread, or dahl.

When the ghee turns a golden yellow and little brown bits of milk solids lie at the bottom of the pan, it is ready to be filtered into a clean jar. Pour it through a fine sieve lined with a coffee filter. Lacking a paper filter, the fine sieve will do. A double sieve is even better. It is not necessary to refrigerate ghee when all the milk solids have been removed, but keep it tightly covered after using.

# To Sprout Whole Beans and Seeds

Use whole lentil beans (gram) or seeds when sprouting. Use 1/2 cup washed lentils. Place them in a covered bowl or jar, set in a warm place, and rinse in tepid water 3 or 4 times a day. They are ready to use when just slightly sprouted, about 24 hours  For cooking purposes use just-sprouted beans, except in Chinese cuisine.

# To Cook Rice

Boil 2 cups water for each cup of washed rice. When water comes to a boil add 1 teaspoon salt and rice (and a tablespoon of ghee for Vata and Pitta cooking). Cover and simmer for 20 minutes. Fluff with a fork before serving.

Or using the same ingredients, place in covered baking dish and bake for 30 minutes at 350°. Fluff immediately and then cover until ready to serve.

## Vata Broth

This basic broth is good as a soup stock, or a gravy and sauce base. When mixed with a quarter teaspoon tamari or soy sauce per cup, it makes a warming boullion drink. As with the other dosha-specific broths, the flavors will change depending on which vata-reducing combination of vegetables and spices you use.

Makes 2 1/2 quarts

2 quarts boiling water
1 teaspoon salt
1/2 teaspoon pepper
Choose at least three different Vata-reducing vegetables, herbs, and spices from this list:
   1 cup carrots, sliced
   1/2 cup tomatoes, chopped
   1/2 cup parsley, chopped
   1/2 cup celery, diced
   1 cup green beans, cut in1-inch pieces
   1 bay leaf
   1/2 teaspoon crushed fenugreek
   1/4 teaspoon crumbled saffron
   1/2 teaspoon ground cumin
   2 tablespoons Vata Churna can be added, or to taste
1 tablespoon ghee

Bring water to a boil in heavy pan. Add the salt, pepper, and vegetables. Simmer covered for 15 minutes. Then add the remaining ingredients. Stir, cover, and simmer another 5 minutes. Then turn off the heat and allow to sit undisturbed half an hour. Strain vegetables and use the broth. The vegetables can be eaten separately with a little salt and pepper and butter.

## Pitta Broth

Pitta broth, a combination of Pitta-reducing vegetables, herbs and spices, is a basic soup stock. The flavor of the broth will vary depending on the combination of ingredients you use. Choose at least three different Pitta-reducing vegetables, herbs, and spices. Pitta broth is useful as a gravy base or for the beginning of a vegetable cream sauce. It is also a refreshing drink for Pitta when served chilled with a celery stick and a garnish of fresh fennel or dill.

Makes 2 quarts

        2 quarts water
        1 cup broccoli, chopped
        1 cup green beans, chopped
        1 cup potatoes, peeled and diced
        1/2 teaspoon salt
        1/4 teaspoon pepper, white or black
        2 tablespoons Pitta Churna
                    or
        2 teaspoons ground coriander
        1/2 teaspoon crushed anise seed
        3 or 4 crushed green cardamom pods
        1 tablespoon ghee (optional)

In a large pot of boiling salted water add vegetables. Turn to low, cover, and simmer for 15 minutes. Stir in remaining ingredients. Cover and simmer 5 more minutes. Then turn off heat and let pot sit undisturbed for 30 minutes. Strain and use the broth. Vegetables can be pureed and used in a creamy soup, or they can be eaten with a little butter.

## Kapha Broth

Makes 2 quarts

2 quarts water
1 teaspoon salt
1/2 teaspoon ground pepper
3 cups Kapha -reducing vegetables --select at least 3 different kinds
1/4 parsley or celery leaves, chopped
2 teaspoons Kapha Churna, or to taste
2 tablespoons mixe fresh herbs--thyme, basil, oregano, marjoram, etc.

Bring water to a boil. Add salt, pepper, parsley, Kapha Churna, and vege-tables--chopping or shredding makes for faster cooking. Cover and bring to a boil. Lower to simmer and sprinkle 2 to 3 teaspoons chopped herbs on top. Stir once, gently. Cover tightly, turn off heat and do not lift lid for 20 to 30 minutes.

## Cornbread

Cornbread is a sweet, salty, hot, light bread that is good for both Kapha and those wanting to reduce weight. It increases Vata a little, and Pitta much more. This is not the best bread choice for Pitta. As with many Kapha-reducing foods, cornbread is good to eat during a light fast, or as part of a light evening meal. Vata should eat this cornbread spread with ghee or butter to help in digestion. Those wanting to lose weight can skip the aditional butter or use very little.

Serves 6 to 8

1 cup white flour
1 cup cornmeal
5 teaspoons baking powder
3/4 teaspoon salt
1 cup milk
2 tablespoons butter or ghee
4 tablespoons sugar

Preheat oven to 375°.

Sift all dry ingredients together except sugar. Heat milk, ghee or butter, and sugar in a saucepan and stir until sugar is dissolved. Then stir into mixed dry ingredients until just moistened. Batter will be thick and a little lumpy. Spread batter in a oiled 9-inch pan and bake for 30 to 35 minutes until light brown.

## French Bread

The taste and crunchy texture is authentically French. This bread, like most plain wheat flour breads, is sweet and good for general nutrition. Eaten in moderation it reduces Vata and Kapha, and is neutral for Pitta. Important note: always eat bread *with* butter for ease of digestion. Vegetables and bread compliment each other. That means they are most efficiently digested when eaten during the same course of the meal.

Makes 2 to 3 loaves.

    2 packages yeast
    3 cups tepid water
    7 1/2 cups unbleached bread flour
    4 teaspoons salt

In a small bowl dissolve the yeast in warm water. In a large bowl mix flour and salt together. Form a well and with a wooden spoon incorporate water and yeast into the flour. Work the flour into a ball by hand, and then transfer to a floured work surface. The dough will feel tacky. Knead dough for about 10 minutes, adding small amounts of flour as necessary. Occasionally throw dough on the work surface. After 10 minutes it will become elastic, but will remain a bit sticky. Grease a large bowl and place dough in it. Cover tightly with plastic wrap. Set in a warm place and allow to double in volume. This will take about 1 1/2 to 2 hours. Punch down, cover, and let rise again. Turn out on a floured surface and knead briefly. Divide into as many loaves as desired. If you are using a French baguette pan, divide the dough into thirds, and make 2 baguettes and 1 oval loaf. Otherwise, two nicely rounded loaves can be made. Place the loaves, covered lightly with a towel, in a warm place and let rise to double volume.

Preheat oven to 425°.

Place a shallow pan of water on the lowest oven shelf. Before putting loaves in oven, slash tops diagonally with razor blade or very sharp knife point. Then spray the loaves with water before placing in oven. Bake on preheated baking tile or on baking sheets sprinkled with a little cornmeal. During the first 18 minutes of baking, open the oven door and spray the loaves with water several times. This will make them very crispy. Then remove the pan of water and finish baking until golden brown. Total baking time is 25-30 minutes.

Remove and cool on wire rack.

## Little Flat Breads

These chewy discs are useful "food pushers" for vegetable dishes, or even as an unusual breakfast bread. Their sweet and slightly bitter tastes decrease Pitta and increase Kapha a little. By substituting sesame seeds for poppy seeds, they will be better for Vata.

Makes 8 small disks

    1 package dry yeast
    1 1/2 cups warm water
    2 tablespoons oil or ghee
    1 teaspoon salt
    1 cup whole wheat flour
    3 to 4 cups white flour
    4 tablespoons poppy seeds

In a large bowl dissolve yeast in warm water. When it is frothy stir in oil, salt, and whole wheat flour. Begin adding white flour, a cup at a time, until a stiff dough is formed. Turn out on a floured surface and wash the bowl.

Oil your hands a little and knead the dough for about 10 minutes, adding small amounts of flour as necessary to make it smooth and elastic. Return the kneaded dough to the bowl. Cover with plastic wrap or a damp towel and place in a warm place to rise. In about an hour to 1 1/2 hours it will be doubled in bulk.

Oil 2 baking sheets. Preheat oven to 450°.

If using sesame seeds, roast them in a heavy skillet over low heat until they are just light brown and starting to pop. Set aside. Do not brown poppy seeds. Turn dough out on clean work surface. Oil your hands. Punch it down and divide into 8 equal parts. Press each part into a circle with a thin middle and higher outer lip. They will look like little pie crusts. Mark the centers a few times with the tines of a fork. Brush with water and sprinkle some seeds on each disk, pressing the seeds lightly into the dough.

Place them, with sides not touching, on baking sheets. Bake 10 minutes or until just brown. They are best when eaten warm.

## Puris and Chapatis

These are fried unleavened breads used in the Indian cuisine for "pushing" the food and sopping up the delectable juices. They are good for everyone, although the sweet and heavy qualities can increase Kapha if too many are eaten. While the ingredients are identical, Chapatis are fried on a hot griddle and Puris, puffy breads, are deep fried in oil.

Makes 15 to 20 Puris or 10 large Chapatis

> 1 1/2 cups whole wheat flour
> 1/2 cup white flour
> 1/2 teaspoon salt
> 1 tablespoon ghee
> 3/4 cup hot water
> 3 to 4 cups oil for frying Puris

In a large bowl stir flours and salt together. Rub in ghee with fingertips until it is evenly combined with flour. Add water and stir into a dough. Add a little more water by teaspoons, if needed, to completely blend all the flour. Knead for 4 or 5 minutes in the bowl. Cover with plastic wrap and allow to rest 1 or 2 hours. The consistency of workable dough should be pliable and firm, but not sticky.

To Make Puris:

Pinch off 1-inch balls of dough, roll in a little flour, then gently roll out on a wooden surface with a rolling pin. Roll in one direction only. Turn the dough over and roll in the opposite direction until it is 4 to 5 inches across and about as thin as a penny, not thinner.

Heat oil in a deep, heavy pan or wok over moderately high heat. When oil is hot gently ease a Puri in so it goes under the surface to the bottom of the pan. When it rises to the top use a pair of tongs and gently push it back under the oil. It should blow up like a balloon. Turn it over in the oil and cook 30 seconds more. Remove and drain on paper towels. Cook each Puri separately and drain.

To Make Chapatis:

Pinch off 2-inch pieces of dough. Roll out evenly and fry on hot greased griddle or heavy skillet for about 30 seconds on each side. Serve immediately.

## Squash Rolls

These tender rolls decrease Vata and Pitta, and increase Kapha. If you have some leftover Ginger Carrot, Curried Squash, or other thick soup, it can be substituted for the cooked squash. These rolls are sweet, oily, and a little heavy.

Makes 1 1/2 dozen

    1/3 cup ghee or butter
    1 cup milk
    1/2 teaspoon crushed saffron
    1/4 teaspoon nutmeg
    1/4 teaspoon  ground cardamom
    1/3 cup brown or white sugar
    1 cup yellow squash, cooked and puréed
    1 package dry yeast
    1/4 cup warm water
    6 to 7 cups unbleached flour

Preheat oven to 375°.

In a saucepan heat ghee, milk, saffron, spices, and sugar. Bring to boiling point. Remove from heat, stir in squash purée. Let cool.

In a large bowl dissolve yeast in very warm water (100°) and wait 2 to 3 minutes for it to foam. Pour in the warm (not hot) squash mixture. Stirr the flour into the squash mixture, a cup at a time, until the dough starts to come away from the sides of the bowl. It will be very soft and tender to the touch.

Turn dough out on floured board, rub your hands with ghee or oil, and knead about 5 minutes until the dough is smooth and not too sticky to handle. Add flour as needed. Let it rest while you wash and oil the bowl. Put the dough in the bowl and turn it to coat with oil. Cover with plastic wrap or a damp towel and let rise in a warm place for 45 minutes to an hour, or until doubled. Push dough down gently and turn out on floured board. Shape golf-ball-size pieces into rolls. Do not stretch them too much to avoid tearing. Place on greased baking sheet. If sides are touching, softer rolls result. Placing rolls 1 inch apart on the sheet makes them crispier. Cover rolls with a damp towel and let rise until doubled (about 40 minutes) or until they are the size you want. Bake 15 to 20 minutes until just golden brown on top. Remove and brush with ghee.

Serve warm.

## Baked Lentil Soup

The idea of "baking" a soup could only originate with a very busy person. It came from Jan Thatcher, who became a new mother when her toddler son seemed to need most of her attention. This extraordinarily neat and easy method of making a delicious dahl is good for everyone, not only new mothers. It's the kind of extremely soupy dahl best for Vata and Kapha to digest. Those following a Pitta-balancing diet might want to double the amount of lentils.

To save time bake rice in a separate covered casserole. Either follow the recipe for Saffron Rice or simply put a cup of rice, 2 cups of water, 1 tablespoon ghee, and salt (to taste) in baking dish. Cover and bake for half an hour. This can be done at the beginning or end of the Baked Lentil Soup's cooking time.

Serves 3 to 4

1/3 cup mung lentils, washed and cleaned
4 cups boiling water
1/2 teaspoon salt
1 teaspoon ghee
1/2 teaspoon Vata Churna
1/2 cup spinach, chopped (optional)
1 teaspoon ghee
1 teaspoon brown mustard seeds
1 teaspoon Vata Churna

Preheat oven to 350°.

Place ingredients in a 1-quart casserole, cover tightly, and bake for 1 1/2 to 2 hours. It will make a very thin lentil dahl.

To prepare spices:

Heat ghee in a small pan over moderate flame. Add mustard seeds and when they start to pop stir in Churna. Add to cooked dahl, stirring well to combine. Serve with rice.

## Creamy Summer Garden Soup

A sweet, slightly bitter, and astringent soup, this is both refreshing in summer and good for reducing Pitta. Because it is cold and heavy this soup increases Vata and Kapha. Use water or Pitta broth as the basic soup stock.

Serves 6 to 8

2 cups Swiss chard, chopped
2 small zucchini,thin sliced
1 cup Bok Choy or Swiss chard leaves, chopped
2 quarts Pitta Broth (see "Other Basics"
1 teaspoon French tarragon, minced
1 tablespoon ghee
1 very ripe avocado, mashed
1 cup heavy cream
1/2 cup shredded raw beets or shredded red cabbage
8 to 10 sprigs fresh fennel or dill

Steam vegetables for 12 minutes or until zucchini is very soft; or cook in pressure cooker for 4 minutes. Cool slightly and puree in food processor or blender until creamy.

Heat Pitta broth in large heavy pot and add vegetable purée. Simmer and stir until well blended. In a separate saucepan heat cream. When just beginning to boil reduce heat and add tarragon, ghee, and mashed avocado. Stir very well and fold into vegetable soup. Cool for an hour, then chill for at least three hours before serving.

Serve in a large decorative glass bowl with shredded beet or cabbage garnish and herbs. Or garnish each bowl individually as you serve.

Note: Recipe can be cut in half if you are cooking for less than 6 persons with Pitta dosha.

## Curried Squash Soup

When served as part of a balanced meal this sweet, salty, slightly pungent soup is good for everyone.

Serves 4 to 6

2 acorn or 1 large butternut squash
2 1/4 cups water or Vata Broth (or broth of choice)
1/2 teaspoon salt
2 tablespoons ghee
1/2 teaspoon ground cumin
1/2 teaspoon cinnamon
1/4 teaspoon ground cardamom
3/4 teaspoon ground ginger
1 cup orange juice (use apple juice for Pitta)

Preheat oven to 400°.

Split squash lengthwise and bake face-down on an oiled tray for 30 minutes to an hour, or until soft. Cool and scoop out the insides. Makes about 3 cups.

Purée in food processor or blender with the water and salt. Pour into 4-quart pan and heat on low flame. In a small pan heat the ghee and sauté the spices. Add to the soup as it is heating. Stir in orange juice and simmer gently, stirring to blend. Serve when steaming hot.

## Ginger Carrot Soup

A pungent, sweet, and salty soup, this is a good appetizer for Vata and can be eaten in moderation by Kapha, but it increases Pitta. This is a great soup for both Kapha and Vata as part of a light meal on a winter-almost-spring day.

Serves 6 to 8

2 cups Vata or Kapha Broth (see "Other Basics")
2 cups milk
2 tablespoons ghee
2 teaspoons sugar
3/4 teaspoon pepper
1/2 teaspoon cardamom
1/4 cup chopped fresh ginger
2 cups shredded carrots
Juice of 1/2 orange
1/2 to 3/4 cup heavy cream
Butter for Vata servings

Bring broth and milk to a boil in a heavy 2-quart pan. Add ghee, sugar, pepper, and cardamom. Stir and cook for a minute over moderately high heat. Add ginger and cook for an additional 2 or 3 minutes until you can smell the ginger clearly. Stir in carrots and orange juice. Cook over low heat, stirring frequently for about an hour until carrots are pulpy. Turn off heat. Cover and let cool.

When ready to serve purée in a food mill or food processor for about 1 minute. Then return to the pot. Reheat just to boiling point and turn to simmer. Add cream. If it seems too thick add a little water. To further enrich the soup for Vata, a pat of butter can be floated on top of each bowl while serving.

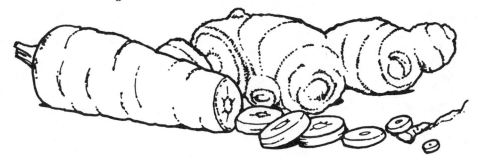

## Khichari

Traditional Indian food for soothing diets. Nutritious and easily digested, Khichari (KITCH-er-ee) is simply rice and dahl cooked so thoroughly together that they make a creamy stew. This makes a good soup for an evening supper or a light meal while fasting. Total cooking time is about 1 1/2 hours.

Serves 2 to 3

1/4 cup mung lentils, cleaned and washed
1 1/2 cup water
1 teaspoon salt
1 teaspoon Vata Churna
1/4 cup rice
2 tablespoons ghee
1 1/4 cup water
1/4 teaspoon saffron (optional)
1 tablespoon ghee
1 teaspoon cumin
1 teaspoon mustard seeds

Bring water to a boil in a 2-quart pan. Add lentils, salt, and Churna. Cover and bring back to a boil, then reduce heat to very low and simmer for about an hour.

Add rice, ghee, water, and saffron. Increase heat and bring to boil again. Then reduce to low and simmer for half an hour. Stir frequently to avoid sticking and add more water if it becomes too thick. Khichari should have the consistency of thick gravy. When ready to serve heat ghee in small pan with spices. When mustard seeds start to pop stir spices into Khichari and serve.

## Masoor Dahl

Dahl (sounds like "doll") is good for people of all body types. For more information about other lentils used in making dahl see Chapter 6, "Something For Everyone." Masoor Dahl is made from coral-colored lentils that cook faster than any others. Although dahl can be flavored with various spice combinations, an easy and most delicious way is by using Maharishi Ayur-Veda Vata Churna. It never fails to produce a rich and authentically Indian dahl.

Serves 4 to 6

    5 cups water
    1 cup red lentils
    1 tablespoon ghee
    1 teaspoon salt, or to taste
    1 tablespoon Vata Churna
                    or
    Choice of ground spices and a pinch of hing (asafoetida)
    2 teaspoons brown mustard seeds
    1 teaspoon ghee or oil

Bring the water to boil in a saucepan. Put the lentils in a shallow dish and pick through them to remove any tiny stones that might be hiding there. Wash the lentils in several changes of cool water until water runs clear. Pour them into the boiling water. Bring back to a boil, lower heat to simmer, and add the salt, ghee, and Vata Churna. Or heat the spices in ghee and add to the cooking lentils. Cover and simmer gently for 20 to 30 minutes, stirring occasionally.

When the lentils are tender and the dahl is a thick soup, fry the mustard seeds in oil or ghee until they just start to pop. It will make a swooshing sound as you add them to the dahl. Serve with a bowl of rice.

## Potage Printanier/French Potato Soup

This is a light, flavorful potato soup in the French style. It takes less than an hour to make and your guests will think it took much longer. Within the context of the whole menu this soup is nourishing for everyone. A steaming bowl of Potage Printanier, a tossed green salad, and a slice of lightly buttered bread makes a good light supper for Kapha types. Tastes in this recipe are sweet, salty, and a little astringent.

Serves 8

2 tablespoons butter or ghee
1 green pepper, chopped
1 1/2 quarts hot water
2 potatoes, pared, quartered, sliced thin
2 carrots, sliced
1/4 cup white rice
6 stalks asparagus, cut in 1/2-inch pieces
1/2 pound spinach, washed and chopped
1 cup light cream
Ground pepper to taste

Melt butter or ghee in a large pot. Add green pepper and sauté until soft. Add water, potatoes, and carrot. Bring to a boil, then reduce to simmer for 15 minutes, stirring occasionally . Add the rice and asparagus. Cover and simmer over very low heat for 25 minutes. Remove the cover and stir in the spinach. Simmer for another 10 minutes. Finally, just before serving add the light cream and just heat through, but do not boil.

**For weight watchers and Kapha:** Decrease to 1 potato, 1/2 cup cream mixed with 1/2 cup water or one cup of skim milk, and 1 tablespoon of butter or ghee.

## Sweet Potato Soup

This soup is a soothing dish to serve as a light meal for those with Vata and Pitta constitutions. It is sweet, heavy, and oily. If made with cream omit the salt.

Serves 4 to 6

6 to 7 cups water
4 medium sweet potatoes
2 carrots (use 1 for Pitta)
1 bay leaf
1/2 to 1 cup heavy cream or half and half
                or
1 cup Vata or Pitta Broth and 1/2 teaspoon salt
2 tablespoons ghee
White pepper, to taste
Cardamom, to taste

Bring water to boil in a large pot. Meanwhile peel and chop potatoes and carrots. When water is boiling add bay leaf, salt, and vegetables. Turn to medium, cover, and cook until soft, or about 40 minutes.

Purée in a food processor or blender until smooth. Return to pot. Add enough cream to make a thin soup, then add ghee, and seasonings to taste. Heat thoroughly and serve.

## Vegetable Soup with Fresh Herbs

This light and pungent soup is excellent for Kapha. It is a highly nutritious and tasty soup that can be enjoyed as an appetizer before a large meal for all body types, although when served by itelf it increases Pitta and Vata slightly.

Serves 6 to 8

2 quarts water
2 teaspoons salt
1 teaspoon coarsely ground pepper
4 cups cauliflower in bite-size pieces
1 large carrot, sliced
1 cup green beans cut in 1-inch pieces
1/4 cup parsley, chopped
1 teaspoon French tarragon, minced, or 1/2 teaspoon dried tarragon
1 to 2 teaspoons minced lemon basil or lemon thyme,
    or
  1 teaspoon dried thyme leaves
3/4 cup tiny semolina pasta or rice

Bring water to a boil. Add salt, pepper, and vegetables. Cover and bring just to a boil. Lower to simmer and sprinkle chopped herbs on top. Stir once, gently. Cover and turn off heat and do not lift lid for 20 to 30 minutes.

When ready to serve, bring pot to a boil and add tiny semolina pasta or rice. Simmer for 8 to 10 minutes and serve.

## Artichokes Stuffed with Herbed Cheese

Available from late winter to early summer, artichokes are at their best and most affordable when most of the popular spring herbs are growing. Fresh herbs impart a superior flavor to this filling. It decreases Vata and Pitta, as do the artichokes. If they were stuffed with Spiced Barley (see page 294 ), then Kapha dieters could enjoy them as well. This dish adds sweet, sour, slightly pungent, cold, heavy, and oily properties to a meal. A pungent appetizer, such as a bowl of hot soup, should precede the meal. And the more varied the bed of herbs and greens used in the salad garnish, the better this dish is for Pitta and Kapha.

Whether served as part of a main meal in springtime or alone as a light evening supper complemented by various condiments, stuffed artichokes are impressive to behold. When individually presented, centered on a large plate, surrounded by torn lettuce, feathery dill and fennel, young purple basil leaves, and a few colorful nasturtium and blue borage flowers, these beautiful artichokes can establish a fine cook's reputation forever.

Serves 4

Prepare the  Artichokes:

> 4 large artichokes
> 1/2 lemon, juiced
> 2 bay leaves (optional)

Bring 2 to 3 quarts of water to a boil in a large pot. Rinse the artichokes and trim the bottom stem even with the bottom leaves. Working from the bottom up, use scissors to clip the sharp pointed leaf tips. Fit the artichokes into the pot of boiling water, add lemon juice and bay leaves. Cover and simmer over moderate heat for 40 minutes. Remove and drain upside down on a rack. Reserve 2 cups of the cooking liquid.

For the Filling:

> 1 1/2 tablespoons ghee
> 1/2 cup sunflower seeds (or other nuts), chopped
> 3 cups soft bread crumbs
> 1 cup parsley, chopped
> 1/2 teaspoon salt
> 1 1/2 cups ricotta or soft panir
> 1 tablespoon grated Parmesan cheese

continues

## Artichokes Stuffed with Herbed Cheese, continued

1/2 cup tofu
1 tablespoon fresh French tarragon, minced
1 tablespoon mixed fresh herbs: thyme, savory, sorrel, mint, basil, etc.
1 teaspoon black pepper
1/2 teaspoon anise seeds, crushed
1/2 teaspoon ground cardamom
2 teaspoons sweet paprika
2 teaspoons olive oil
4 or 5 whole allspice

For Garnish:

Lettuce varieties, fennel, dill, tarragon, basil; orange, pineapple, or lemon mint; chive blossoms, edible flowers.

Heat ghee in a large pot over moderate heat. Stir in seeds and fry until light brown, about 2 minutes. Add bread crumbs, parsley, and salt. Toss well until mixed. Cover and set aside while preparing cheese mixture.

In a large bowl mash the cheeses and tofu together. Using a mortar and pestle crush the spices and herbs together in the olive oil. Form a thick paste (pesto). Mix the cheese and pesto thoroughly together, and then combine with the bread crumbs.

Stuff the Artichokes:

Set the artichokes upright and carefully open each one until the center choke is exposed. Pull this out with your fingers or use the tip of a sharp knife to get started. Place a large spoonful of filling in the center. Then slip some between all the leaves except the outer ones. Divide the filling equally among the artichokes. When thoroughly stuffed, tie each with a cotton string or ribbon to hold them together. Pour 1 cup of reserved liquid and allspice in a large pot. Lay metal or bamboo steamer flat in the pot. Gently set the artichokes on the steamer so the sides touch. Cover and simmer over low for 20 minutes. If liquid evaporates before time is up, add more. Remove from pot and allow to sit for 15 minutes before handling. Cut strings. Set each artichoke on a bed of lettuce and decorate with herbs and flowers. Serve warm.

## Baked Wild Rice Casserole

Although wild rice, seed of a native north American aquatic grass, is not truly a rice it has similar properties. Because it is a thicker and rougher grain it takes longer to cook than other rice and can be eaten in greater quantities by those following a Kapha diet.

Serves 4 to 6

1 tablespoon ghee or butter
1/4 cup celery, thinly sliced
1 cup wild rice, washed
2 cups vegetable broth (Vata, Pitta, or Kapha)
      or
  2 cups water and 2 teaspoons Kapha Churna
1/2 teaspoon salt
1 teaspoon ghee or butter
1 tablespoon sliced almonds
1 tablespoon ghee or olive oil
1/2 cup chopped sweet red pepper
1/2 cup carrots, shredded
1/2 teaspoon salt

Preheat oven to 350°.

Melt one tablespoon of butter in heavy casserole over moderate heat. Add celery and wild rice frying until well-coated. Pour broth over rice and sprinkle on salt. Bring just to a boil, then cover tightly and bake in middle of oven for 1 hour. Remove and rest without uncovering for 15 minutes. Meanwhile in small heavy pan melt a teaspoon of butter and brown the almonds. Set aside. Then heat the remaining ghee in a skillet, add the red peppers and salt, tossing well until the peppers are limp.

To serve, toss peppers andcarrots with the rice. Sprinkle almonds on top.

**For those reducing weight:** Omit almonds and reduce ghee and oil by one half.

## Curried Vegetables and Panir

A simple mixture of mixed spiced vegetables, and crisply fried panir served on a bed of Basmati or other long grain white rice, this dish is a basic standby that can be made for any constitutions by using the appropriate blend of vegetables and spices. When cooking for a group with varied needs, use many different vegetables so everyone has several to choose. This recipe is just an example of proportions and cooking methods. Substitute whatever fresh, seasonally available vegetables you prefer for your individual diet.

Serves 4 to 6

1 1/2 tablespoons ghee
1 1/2 cups 1-inch panir cubes (see "Other Basics" for recipe)
2 tablespoons sunflower or safflower oil
1 cup sweet potato, diced
2 stalks celery, sliced
1 carrot, thinly sliced
2 stems broccoli, chopped
1 medium turnip, diced
1 cup green beans, in 1-inch pieces
1 medium tomato, peeled and cut in wedges
1/4 cup raisins
1/2 teaspoon salt
2 teaspoons ghee or oil
1 teaspoon ground coriander
1/2 teaspoon ground cumin
1/2 teaspoon ground fenugreek
1/2 teaspoon ground cardamom
1 1/2 cups water

Heat ghee in a large, heavy skillet over moderately high heat. Add panir cubes and allow to fry without turning for 3 or 4 minutes. When slightly crispy turn to another side. Continue frying until all sides are richly browned. Remove from pan and set aside. In the same skillet heat the 2 tablespoons of oil. Add vegetables, one kind at a time. Fry each for 2 minutes, stirring well, before adding the next ingredient.

## Curried Vegetables and Panir, continued

When all the vegetables and raisins have been added, push everything to the sides of the pan to make a small well in the center. Pour in 2 teaspoons ghee and sprinkle in the mixed ground spices. Stir until heated, then blend with all the vegetables. Add the panir and pour the water over everything, cover tightly, and turn the flame to low. Allow to simmer, covered for 15 minutes. Serve on a bed of hot rice.

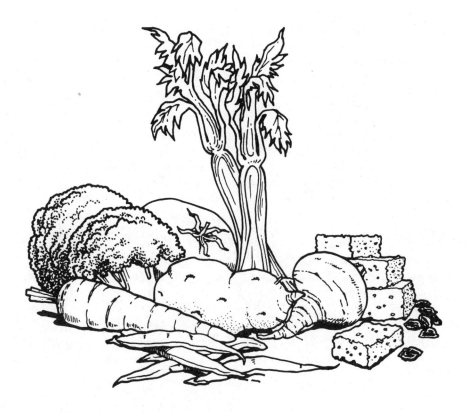

## Green and Gold Baked Squash

With predominantly astringent, bitter, slightly sour, and slightly pungent tastes and hot, light, and slightly oily qualities, this colorful main dish is a good choice for reducing Kapha.  Vata or Pitta may have a small amount as part of a balanced meal, but only as a side dish.  Allow 1/2 squash per serving.  You can either stuff each half separately, or peel squash, cut into 2-inch cubes, and mix in an oiled baking pan with the stuffing.

Serves 4

> 2 acorn or trimmed butternut squash
> 2 teaspoons ghee
> 1/2 teaspoon turmeric
> 1/2 teaspoon ground thyme
> 1 teaspoon licorice root powder
> 1 teaspoon fresh ginger, shredded (reduce for Pitta)
> > or
> 1/4 teaspoon ground ginger
> 1/2 cup skim milk ricotta
> 1 cup cooked millet ( use cooked rice for Vata)
> 1 cup fresh spinach, washed and chopped fine
> 1 medium Granny Smith, Greening, or other tart apple, diced
> 1 teaspoon nutmeg
> 1 cup hot water

Preheat oven to 375°.

Heat the ghee in a small heavy pan over moderately high heat.  Add the turmeric, thyme, licorice root, and ginger.  Stir in the ricotta with a sharp chopping motion and just blend together. Toss with the millet, spinach, and diced apple.  Pile stuffing into the squash and set in a 9 x 12 inch oiled pan. Pour water around squash.  Cover tightly and bake for 45 minutes or until the squash is tender when pierced with a fork.

## Green Beans in Tomato Sauce
## (Fagioloni in Umido Volponi)

A delicious main dish, this has properly balanced tastes and qualities that reduce all doshas. It is pleasantly sweet and salty. The green beans must be very well cooked to balance Vata.

Serves 4

1 pound fresh green beans
1 pound ripe tomatoes, or a 14-ounce can of tomatoes, chopped
2 tablespoons olive oil or vegetable oil
1/2 teaspoon each of oregano, thyme, and basil
Salt and pepper to taste

Wash, de-string, and cut beans into 1-inch pieces. Blanch and peel fresh tomatoes, then chop.

Heat the oil in a 2-quart saucepan. Add beans, tomatoes, and crushed herbs. Stir a few times, then add salt and pepper to taste. Cover and simmer over low heat for about 45 minutes, until the beans are quite tender and the tomatoes saucy. If the sauce starts to stick, add a little water during cooking. Serve hot with pasta.

## Layered Vegetable Loaf

Lightly breaded eggplant slices layered with a variety of Kapha-decreasing vegetables in a loaf pan makes this entree light in quality with the astringent, bitter, pungent, and slightly sour tastes good for Kapha diets.   It can be eaten as it is by Vata and Pitta types as a side dish.   Otherwise use the sliced eggplant layered with Vata-or Pitta-decreasing vegetables and herbs.

Makes 1 loaf


1 medium eggplant
1 1/2 cups fine bread crumbs
3 tablespoons cream
1 tablespoon olive oil
1 teaspoon fresh basil, minced ( or 1/2 teaspoon dried)
1 teaspoon fresh oregano, minced ( or 1/2 teaspoon dried)
1/2 teaspoon black pepper
1/2 teaspoon salt
1 cup shredded carrots
1 cup peas, steamed
1 cup spinach or chard, chopped
2 tablespoons red sweet pepper, diced
1/4 cup celery leaves, chopped
1 medium tomato, peeled, seeded, thinly sliced
1/4 cup roasted sunflower seeds, chopped
1/2 cup water


Preheat oven to 350°.

Peel eggplant and cut 10 to12 slices 1/2-inch thick.  Put cream in a shallow bowl, dip each slice in cream and then in bread crumbs.  Tightly fit a layer of breaded eggplant on the bottom of the pan.  Mix the remaining ingredients together, except the tomato and sunflower seeds, and pat a third of the mixture on the eggplant.  Lay a couple of tomato slices on top.  Make 3 such layers, ending with eggplant.  Sprinkle chopped seeds on top.  Pour on water.  Cover tightly and bake  45 minutes.  Let the loaf rest 10 minutes before slicing.

## Lightly Seasoned Vegetables

Vegetables prepared this way make a good side dish or a light evening meal
for anyone following a Vata-reducing diet or any children who like mixed
vegetables.

Serves 4 to 6

1 cup potatoes, diced
1/2 cup carrots, sliced thin
1/2 cup beets, sliced thin
1 cup yellow squash, sliced thin
1/2 cup (or more to taste) spinach, chopped
2 tablespoons ghee
1/2 teaspoon brown mustard seeds
1/2 teaspoon cardamom, ground
1 teaspoon Vata Churna
      or
 1/2 teaspoon cumin, ground
8 fenugreek seeds, ground

Cook vegetables in a pressure cooker or steamer until tender. In a large
skillet heat the ghee and mustard seeds. When the seeds start to pop add
the remaining spices and salt. Stir for 30 seconds and then add the
vegetables. Sauté for about 2 minutes or until well coated with the spices.

**For Pitta and Kapha:** Follow the same instructions but substitute Pitta-
or Kapha-reducing vegetables and spices.

## Moroccan Delight

An elaborate and beautiful dish to serve at a party, this recipe reduces Pitta and Vata and increases Kapha (although it is nourishing for Kapha). The "delight" is in savoring a variety of stimulating flavors and exotic color combinations. By preparing groups of ingredients separately, the tastes remain distinct from one another even after they are finally  combined before serving. A little of every taste is represented, but it is mostly sweet in taste and heavy and oily in quality.

Serves 4 to 6 generously

> 2 cups marinated tofu (see following recipe)
> 2 cups broccoli flowerets
> 2 cups cauliflowerets
> 1 large sweet pimento pepper, cut in bite-size pieces
> 1  can (8 ounces) artichoke hearts, not marinated, quartered
> Ghee
> 2 tablespoons olive oil, or other cooking oil
> 1/2 cup warm water
> 1/2 teaspoon ground coriander
> 1 tablespoon turmeric
> 1 teaspoon ground cardamom
> 1/2 teaspoon to 1 teaspoon salt, to taste
> 1/2 cup bright orange dried apricots, sliced
> 1/4 cup pitted dates, chopped
> 6 cups cooked couscous or rice
> 1/4 cup blanched almonds, sliced

Prepare Marinated Tofu in Advance:

Marinate tofu at least 2 hours before you are ready to cook. Use firm tofu with the water pressed out, or frozen, thawed, and squeezed for more texture.

> 1 quart sweet red fruit juice, such as raspberry, pomegranate, plum, strawberry, or a blend of these
> 1/4 teaspoon each nutmeg, ground coriander, and cinnamon
> 1 tablespoon tamari
> 1 pound tofu—with water pressed out and cubed

## Moroccan Delight continued

In a 2 quart-saucepan heat the juice, spices, and tamari. Remove from heat and mix in the tofu cubes. Cover and marinate for two or three hours at room temperature, or overnight in the refrigerator. Or for a quick marinade omit the spices and simply pour juice and tamari mixture over the tofu. Cover and set aside for at least two hours. When ready to prepare, drain the tofu.

Steam broccoli and cauliflower for 10 minutes. Set aside.

To Prepare:

Heat 3 tablespoons ghee in a wok or heavy frying pan and sauté tofu cubes until they are lightly browned—about 10 minutes. Set aside in a large bowl. In the same pan heat 1 tablespoon of ghee over medium heat. Add sesame seeds and stir until they begin to turn brown and start popping. Turn heat to high and immediately add red pepper pieces and artichoke hearts. Sauté for 1 minute, tossing to cover the vegetables with the seeds. Then gently mix in with the tofu. Set aside and cover.

Again in the same pan heat 2 tablespoons of oil over medium heat. Add turmeric, coriander, cardamom, and salt. Stir until turmeric lumps disappear. Then slowly stir in 1/2 cup warm water. This makes a golden sauce. Add steamed broccoli and cauliflower. Stir until cauliflower is uniformly golden, then add apricots and dates. Add more water as needed to keep the sauce from drying out. Simmer over low heat for another minute, stirring frequently. Then gently fold in the tofu cubes and stir-fry another minute or 2 until they are dark brown. Arrange on a bed of steaming couscous or rice and sprinkle with almonds.

If not serving immediately, cover tightly and keep warm in 200° oven.

To prepare this dish for a celebration or large party allow 1/2 cup tofu and 1/2 cup vegetables per person. For an authentic ethnic touch serve with Little Flat Breads or pita bread.

## Couscous

Couscous can be served with any vegetable dish or as a rice substitute. Made from semolina flour, it is a sweet-tasting addition to any meal and is good for decreasing Vata and Pitta, and increasing Kapha a little. Whole wheat couscous, available at natural food stores, is more nourishing than the creamy yellow variety, but not as light and fluffy.

Serves 4 to 6

4 cups water
2 cups couscous
2 tablespoons oil or ghee
1 teaspoon salt

Add the couscous to boiling water. When it comes to a second boil add the oil and salt, and stir vigorously with a wooden spoon until all the water evaporates and it is steamy, almost sizzling. Then remove from heat and cover. Let stand for 10 to 15 minutes. Before serving fluff with a fork. While it is standing, you can sauté some vegetables to serve with it.

## Fast Couscous—The Oven Method

2 cups couscous
1 tablespoon ghee or light oil
1 teaspoon salt
4 cups boiling water
Preheat oven to 400°.

Spread couscous in a 2-quart glass or ovenproof casserole. Add ghee or oil and sprinkle with salt. Pour boiling water over the couscous. Seal tightly with aluminum foil and a lid. Bake for 20 minutes. Remove the foil and fluff with a fork while steamy.

## Oven Baked French Fries

French Fries are so heavy, oily, and fat increasing that Kapha should eat less of them. French fries decrease Vata, are neutral for Pitta, and increase Kapha.

1 potato per person
1/2 tablespoon butter per person
Salt and pepper to taste

Preheat oven to 350°.

Slice potatoes in long thin "frenched" shapes. Melt the butter and coat the potatoes. Arrange them on baking sheets 1 or 2 layers thick. Bake for at least 1 hour, turning the potatoes after about 30 minutes. They are done when they turn golden brown. For large amounts (more than 5 potatoes ) baking may take longer.

## Pasta and Green Sauce

The green herbs make this sauce a flavorful accompaniment to spaghetti or linguini. When served with pasta this dish decreases Vata, is neutral for Pitta, and increases Kapha. Kapha can eat more of this as a main dish if cooked barley is substituted for the pasta. Parmesan cheese can be used by both Vata and Kapha. The combined qualities of this recipe are sweet, salty, oily, and heavy.

Serves 3-4

1 cup minced parsley
3/4 cup minced fresh basil or 1/2 cup dried crushed basil
1 teaspoon salt
1/2 cup chopped nuts—pine nuts are best
1/2 cup olive oil
Grated parmesan cheese, optional

Grind herbs, salt, and nuts in mortar and pestle, or chop in a food processor with a steel blade. Add the oil and combine until smooth. This makes about 1 1/2 cups of simple "pesto." Cook spaghetti or other pasta according to package directions. Drain and toss with green sauce.

281

## Peas Braised with Lettuce
## ( Pois Braise Laitue)

This French dish is a delightful blend of sweet and sour tastes.  It combines consistency with the refreshing lightness of spring vegetables and makes a satisfying entree served with Rice Pilaf.  The recipe has a  neutral effect on Vata and Pitta doshas and increases Kapha slightly.

Serves 4 to 6

> 1 firm Boston lettuce
> 3 sprigs each:
>> parsley
>> thyme
>> marjoram
> 2 tablespoons butter
> 1 pepper—red bell or pimento, diced or chopped
> 2 cups fresh peas
> 1 cup chopped spinach
> 1/2 cup water
> 1/2 teaspoon salt
> 1/2 teaspoon sugar

Wash lettuce and cut into 4 to 6 wedges.  Tie each wedge together with cotton string to keep its shape.  Tie herb sprigs together.  In a heavy 3-quart saucepan put all the ingredients except 2 tablespoons of butter.  Bring to a boil over moderate heat, tossing lightly.  Cover the pan and cook over low heat for 30 minutes, stirring frequently until vegetables are tender and the liquid is cooked away.  Remove the herbs and the strings from the lettuce wedges.  Add 2 tablespoons butter, toss, and serve on a bed of rice.

Note: Sugar and butter can be reduced by half for Kapha and others watching their weight.

## Quick Vegetable Medley

A colorful sweet, oily, slightly pungent Vata-decreasing dish that is very easy to make. Serve with rice or couscous.

Serves 4


2 tablespoons ghee
1/2 teaspoon ground cumin
1 teaspoon Vata Churna
1/2 teaspoon salt
1 medium cucumber, peeled, seeded, diced
1 cup shredded beets
1 cup shredded carrots


Heat ghee in a skillet over a moderate flame. Stir in spices and vegetables. Cover and reduce heat to low. Stir frequently frying until vegetables are well cooked and soft.

## Rich Stuffed Peppers

A delicious main dish that is nourishing for Vata  with its sweet, salty, bitter, and slightly astringent tastes.  Kapha would eat little of ththis dish. This warm, rich, heavy stuffing can be baked separately in a buttered casserole and served as a side dish for Pitta and Vata.

Serves 6

3 large green peppers, halved and blanched
1/2 cup ghee or butter
3/4 cup celery stalks and leaves, chopped
2 small zucchini, cubed
1/4 cup parsley, chopped
1/2 cup sweet red pepper, chopped
1/4 cup pecans or cashews, coarsely chopped
4 cups soft bread cubes
1/2 teaspoon salt
1 teaspoon crushed sage
1/2 teaspoon thyme
1/4  to 1/2 teaspoon coarsely ground pepper

To Blanch Peppers:

Bring 2 quarts of water to a  boil. Meanwhile halve peppers and remove seeds and membrane. Drop them into boiling water and allow to boil for 3 minutes. Remove from pot and immediately run under cold water. Drain with hollow side down on a towel until ready to stuff.

Preheat oven to 350°.

For the Stuffing:

Heat ghee in a large frying pan or deep pot.  Add vegetables and sauté, stirring frequently for about 20 minutes or until soft.  Add nuts, then the bread cubes and seasonings.  Toss well and heat through.  Mound stuffing into pepper halves and place in lightly oiled 9 x12 inch baking pan.  Bake uncovered for 10 minutes.

## Simply Baked Carrots

This simply made side dish is nourishing for a Vata. By reducing the ghee to 1 tablespoon it makes a good side dish for Kapha.

Serves 2 to 3

1/2 pound carrots
1/4 cup water
1/4 teaspoon salt
4 tablespoons ghee
1/4 cup sesame seeds

Preheat oven to 350°.

Julienne carrots or cut into narrow finger-length pieces. Place in saucepan with water and salt. Boil over moderately high flame just until tender. test with a fork. Arrange carrots in a small deep baking pan, pour in any remaining liquid along with them. Sprinkle with sesame seeds and ghee. Bake, uncovered, for 30 minutes or until golden brown and baste several times with juices.

## Simple Rice Pilaf

This easy dish to make adds sweet and salty tastes to the meal. It is best served with steamed or sautéed vegetables. As part of a balanced meal it is good for everyone.

Makes about 2 cups

3 tablespoons ghee or butter
1 stalk celery, chopped
1 cup white rice
1/2 teaspoon basil, crushed,
            or
   1 teaspoon fresh basil, chopped
1 tablespoon parsley, chopped
1/2 teaspoon salt
1/2 teaspoon  pepper, or to taste
2  cups water

Melt ghee in a 2-quart saucepan and sauté celery . Add rice and cook about one minute until rice is transparent. Ghee should just cover rice. Add basil, parsley, salt, and pepper. Then add water. Bring to boil, reduce to low heat, and simmer covered tightly for about 20 minutes or until all the water is absorbed.  Fluff and serve.

For Pitta: Omit the basil and increase the parsley to taste.

## Spicy Vegetable Curry

This Spicy Vegetable Curry decreases Kapha and Vata, and increases Pitta somewhat. It makes a good side dish for Pitta when served as part of a meal with other Pitta-reducing selections. The predominant tastes are pungent, sour, sweet, slightly bitter, and astringent with hot, oily qualities. This combination makes it a good main dish anytime for those following a Kapha-reducing diet.

Wash, peel, chop, and grind all the ingredients before beginning to cook. Select fresh, seasonally available vegetables. If you omit those vegetables not available listed in this recipe, be sure to substitute others in the correct quantity to make up the total amount called for. Although fresh vegetables are always the best choice, buying good quality fresh tomatoes, peas, and other summer favorites might not be practical in winter. The occasional use—once every week or two—of canned or frozen ingredients is all right as long as they make up a small part of the recipe.

Serves 6 to 8

Prepare Vegetables:

4 medium carrots, sliced
4 small zucchini, sliced thin
1 1/2 cups green beans, cut in 1/2-inch pieces
1/2 cup peas, fresh or frozen
1 small cauliflower, broken into flowerets
1 small eggplant, peeled and diced
3 to 4 medium tomatoes, skinned and diced
or
1 18-ounce can peeled tomatoes, chopped in blender or food processor

For the Curry:

3 tablespoons ghee
1 tablespoon Kapha Churna, or more to taste
1 teaspoon salt
1/2 cup water, or more as needed
3 tablespoons olive oil, or other cooking oil
1 teaspoon turmeric
3/4 teaspoon ground cumin

continues

## Spicey Vegetable Curry continued

In a Large Pot:

Heat 3 tablespoons ghee over moderate heat. Add Kapha Churna, stir briefly, then add carrots and zucchini slices. Turn heat to low and stir until well-coated with ghee. Cover and allow to simmer for 3 minutes. Add green beans, peas, salt, and 1/2 cup water. Cover and continue simmering on low while preparing the other ingredients.

In a Frying Pan or Large Wok:

Heat 2 tablespoons oil over moderately high heat. Add turmeric and cumin. Mix well together for about 30 seconds, then stir in cauliflower. Stir fry about 2 minutes or until cauliflower is evenly coated and bright gold. Push cauliflower to the sides of the pan and add 1 tablespoon of oil to the center. When it is hot stir in eggplant. Cook 1 minute. Then mix tomatoes in with the eggplant and cauliflower. Stir until everything is well blended. It should become very liquid, like a tomato sauce. If not, add water gradually. Cover and turn heat to low and simmer 3 to 4 minutes.

About 10 minutes before serving stir the tomato mixture into the large pot. Mix gently and simmer on low. Serve with rice.

Note: If any curry is left after the meal, save it until evening and heat it by frying in hot oil. Then stuff it in folded chapatis, tortillas, or pita bread. Serve these with a tossed salad for a light meal.

## Stuffed Shells and Artichoke Cream Sauce

Easily made, this elegant entree is best for Vata and Pitta. Kapha would eat a small portion of this sweet, oily, heavy, slightly sour, slightly pungent dish.

Serves 4  Allow 3 shells per serving.

12 large pasta shells
1 tablespoon olive oil or ghee
1 tablespoon basil pesto (see Green Sauce, page 281)
2 cups heavy cream
1/4 cup Parmesan cheese, grated
1 can artichoke hearts, drained and quartered
1 medium sweet red pepper, cut in 1-inch pieces

Cook pasta shells in a large pot of boiling salted water for 10 minutes. Drain and run under cold water to cool. Prepare the sauce while shells cook. In a heavy 2-quart sauce pan heat the oil, add the pesto and peppers. Fry until peppers are soft. Add cream and stir in cheese. Simmer until bubbling and slightly thickened. Cover and stuff the shells.

Preheat oven to 400°.

For the stuffing:

1 cup soft tofu
1 cup ricotta
1 cup chopped parsley
1/2 cup chopped spinach
1 teaspoon black or white pepper
1/2 teaspoon nutmeg

Mix all the ingredients together and stuff each cooled shell. Pour a spoonful of sauce in the bottom of a 8-inch square baking pan. Arrange the stuffed shells closely together and fill in the spaces with quartered artichoke hearts. Sprinkle with paprika and a little grated Parmesan, if you like. Cover and bake for 30 minutes.

## Sweet Summer Curry

This is sweet and unctuous, astringent, warm, heavy, and a little salty that makes a good main dish for Pitta and Vata. Kapha can eat very moderately of this curry. The more pungent ones suit Kapha better. By increasing the spinach and decreasing the raisins, grapes and potatoes this sweet curry would make a better side dish for Kapha types. The Fried-Spiced Potatoes is a Kapha side dish also.

When preparing sprouted lentils for frying, soak them in warm water, cover, and allow to sit overnight or just long enough for the sprouts to begin coming out. Wash them well in cool water before using.

Serves 4 to 6 generously

Prepare Fried-Spiced Potatoes and allow them to steam while you cook the fruits and vegetables.

## Fried-Spiced Potatoes

1/4 cup light oil, safflower or sunflower
1/2 teaspoon nutmeg
1/2 teaspoon ground cardamom
1/2 teaspoon coriander
4 medium red-skinned potatoes, scrubbed and diced
1/2 teaspoon salt
1/2 cup warm water

In a heavy frying pan heat oil over medium high heat. Add nutmeg, cardamom, and coriander. Stir in potatoes. When they are coated with oil and spices sprinkle with salt. Fry over moderate heat, stirring frequently, for 10 minutes. Pour in water, cover, and simmer on low heat for 5 minutes. Turn off heat and leave covered until ready to combine with remaining ingredients.

To Curry Vegetables and Fruits:

4 to 6 tablespoons ghee
1/2 teaspoon brown mustard seeds (or poppy seeds for Pitta, if desired)
2 tablespoons Pitta Churna
1 cup sprouted whole urad lentils (Indian black gram)

## Sweet Summer Curry   continued

2 apples, peeled and diced
2 medium yellow summer squash, diced
3/4 teaspoon salt
1/2 cup raisins
1/2 cup seedless grapes, green or red
1 cup  sweet fruit juice: pineapple-coconut, papaya, mango, or white
    grape
3/4 cup fried coconut
1/2 cup spinach, washed and chopped

In a large frying pan or wok heat 2 tablespoons ghee over medium high heat. Add mustard seeds (or poppy seeds). When seeds begin to pop add Pitta Churna. Stir 1 minute. Add sprouts. Cook 2 to 3 minutes, stirring frequently. Push the sprouts to the sides of the pan and add 2 more table-spoons of ghee in the center. When  ghee is hot, add chopped apples  and squash. Stir in salt. Cook, stirring gently, for 3 to 4 minutes, then mix together with the sprouts. Add raisins, grapes, and fruit juice. Cover and simmer on low for 10 minutes. Gently toss in fried potatoes and mix well. Stir in 1/2 cup toasted coconut. Reserve 1/4 cup for garnish. Spread spinach evenly on top and sprinkle with remaining coconut.  Cover.  Turn off heat and let steam for 10 minutes.

Serve on a platter of Saffron Rice or plain rice for Pitta in hot weather.

## To Fry Coconut

Heat 2 tablespoons ghee in a small pan over moderate heat. Add coconut and toss well to coat. Heat slowly, stirring constantly until light brown. Remove from heat and set aside.

## Saffron Rice

Rice is cold, sweet, and heavy. It reduced Vata and Pitta, and increases Kapha. But this is a good way to prepare rice for Kapha types because the saffron is a heating herb; and by frying the rice in a little oil before boiling it becomes less heavy. Vata types can use the heat of saffron, but the rice does not need to be fried first. Those with Pitta constitutions do not need to lighten the rice by frying either. Saffron can be eaten in moderation by Pitta in cold months.

Baking rice makes in a casserole is easy and makes dependably fluffy rice.

Makes 2 cups

2 cups boiling water
1/2 teaspoon salt
1 cup washed Basmati rice, or other long grain white rice
3/4 teaspoon saffron
2 tablespoons ghee

Preheat oven to 350°.

Heat 1 tablespoon ghee in frying pan over moderate heat. Add washed rice and stir to coat. Fry 3 to 4 minutes. Pour water, salt, and saffron into a 2-quart casserole. Stir in ghee. Spread rice evenly on the bottom. Cover tightly with foil and bake for 30 minutes. Fluff with a fork when done, and again before serving.

## Tofu Nut Burgers

A good main dish that is both sweet and nourishing, tofu nut burgers have a tonic (healthfully nourishing) effect. They are a body-building food that decreases Vata, is neutral for Pitta, and increases Kapha. When eaten with the usual selection of condiments—pickles, olives, mustard, catsup, and so forth—they are more easily digested. Choose from condiments according to taste.

Makes 8 burgers

  1 pound tofu
  2 cups cooked brown rice
  1 cup ground nuts—medium grind
  3 tablespoons tamari, or to taste
  1 stalk of celery, chopped and sautéed

Preheat oven to 350°.

Combine tofu with 1 1/2 cups brown rice in a food processor, blending thoroughly. Add remaining ingredients, mix, and form into patties. Bake on greased baking sheet for 25 to 35 minutes. A nice brown crust will form on the outside but they will stay moist on the inside.

Serve hot, or save and reheat by putting in 350° oven for 5 minutes.

Tofu burgers can be baked at the same time as the Oven-Baked French Fries.

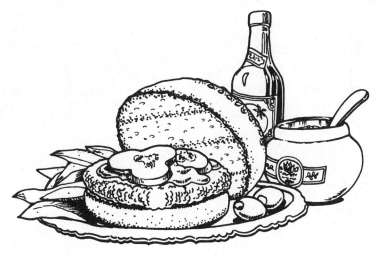

## Vegetables with Spiced and Roasted Barley

Everyone can eat this dish as part of a balanced meal, but it is a first choice for Kapha, and good to eat on light fasting days.  The outstanding tastes of this recipe are pungent, sweet, and salty.  It should be served as a side dish rather than the main course for Vata and Pitta. By substituting cooked brown rice for the barley, it would make a more substantial main dish for thin people.

Serves 6 to 8

To prepare the barley:

    3 tablespoons ghee
    1/2 teaspoon cayenne
    1 cup barley, rinsed
    1 1/2 teaspoons salt
    31/2 cups hot water

Heat ghee in a heavy skillet or 2-quart pot over moderate heat.  Stir in the cayenne. After one minute stir in barley. Roast barley by continuously stirring until grains are medium brown. Watch carefully not to burn it. Then sprinkle on salt, add hot water, and stir once or twice. Cover tightly and simmer for about 1 hour. It's all right if some liquid remains. Fluff up and set aside while you prepare vegetables. Or make ahead and prepare vegetables just before serving.

To prepare the vegetables:

    1 cup broccoli, cut in flowerets
    2 tablespoons olive oil
    1 teaspoon minced fresh ginger or 1/2 teaspoon ground ginger
    1/4 cup sesame seeds
    1/4 cup roasted pumpkin seeds
    1 sweet red pepper, cut in 1-inch squares
    1 cup Swiss chard (mixed ruby and white look best)—washed and chopped
    1/2 cup beet greens, washed and chopped
    2 teaspoons salt
    1/2 teaspoon coarsely ground pepper

## Vegetables with Spiced and Roasted Barley, continued

Steam broccoli for 3 to 4 minutes and set aside. Heat the oil in a wok or large heavy frying pan. Add ginger and sesame seeds. Fry over moderate heat until seeds start to pop. Add half the pumpkin seeds, stir, add red peppers, stir; and add chard and beet greens. Add steamed broccoli, salt, and pepper. Toss well and cover. Turn off heat and let vegetables steam while you reheat the barley over medium heat until any remaining liquid is gone. Stir in remaining 1/4 cup pumpkin seeds and spread the barley on serving platter. Arrange the vegetables on the bed of barley and serve.

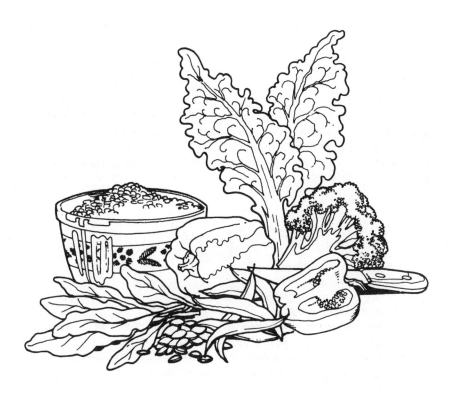

## Vegetable Whole Grain Sauté

Anyone can enjoy this recipe as part of a balanced meal. It's a light, easily-digested main dish that is just right for Kapha when barley is used. Bulgar, cracked wheat, or brown rice are better whole grains for those following Pitta and Vata diets. This recipe adds sweet, astringent tastes, and light and oily qualities to the complete menu. Even when prepared with cooked barley it can be served to anyone as the main part of a light meal. The use of sprouted urad beans—whole black gram—adds a sweet, nutty flavor. These sprouts are very nourishing and somewhat weight producing. They are especially useful for Vata and Pitta diets. For those who are reducing weight mung bean or brown lentil sprouts can be used instead of the more fattening urad.

Serves 4

If made with barley:

> 2 cups water
> 3/4 cup barley, pearled or hulled
> 1/2 teaspoon salt
> 2 teaspoons olive oil

In a heavy 1-quart pan bring water to a boil. Add salt and rinsed barley. Cover and simmer gently for 40 minutes until the barley is soft but is still holding its shape. When cooked, toss with olive oil, cover, and set aside until ready to serve.

For bulgar or cracked wheat:

> 2 cups water
> 1 cup bulgar or cracked wheat
> 2 teaspoons olive oil

Bring water to a boil. Place bulgar in a 1-quart bowl. Pour water over. Cover and set aside for about 15 or 20 minutes until the bulgar is tender. Drain any excess water. Pour on olive oil and toss with a fork. Cover until ready to serve.

## Vegetable Whole Grain Sauté, continued

For the vegetables:

  2 teaspoons sesame oil
  2 tablespoons sunflower seeds
  1/2 teaspoon salt
  1/2 teaspoon coarsely ground pepper
  1/2 cup shredded zucchini
  3/4 cup shredded carrots
  1/2 cup minced celery
  1 cup urad beans, sprouted (see "Other Basics")

Heat sesame oil in large wok or large heavy frying pan over medium high heat. Add sunflower seeds, salt, and pepper and sauté about 1 minute or until seeds are just browning. Add zucchini and carrots and toss with seeds, frying for about a minute. Then add minced celery and sprouts, and cook another minute. Turn off heat, cover, and prepare barley or bulgar for serving.

Before serving:

  1/2 teaspoon olive oil
  1 teaspoon crushed sage
  2 teaspoons fresh thyme, minced
          or
  1/2 teaspoon dried thyme, crushed
  Lemon wedges

In a heavy frying pan heat 1/2 teaspoon olive oil. Add cooked barley, sage, and thyme, mixing well and heat thoroughly. Mound on a serving plate with an indentation in the center. Pile the sautéed vegetables on top. Decorate with lemon wedges.

## Zucchini and Tomato Fry

A satisfying and colorful main dish with sweet, sour, bitter, salty, and slightly pungent tastes, this dish can be enjoyed by Vata, and in moderation by Kapha. It increases Pitta.

Serves 4

> 2 tablespoons ghee
> 1 teaspoon black mustard
> 1 teaspoon cumin seeds, roasted and crushed
> 1 teaspoon coriander, ground
> 1/4 teaspoon fenugreek, ground
> 1 teaspoon turmeric
> 1/2 teaspoon ground ginger
> 4 medium zucchini, peeled, quartered, and sliced thin
> 2 to 3 tomatoes, peeled and sliced
> 1/2 teaspoon salt (or to taste)

Heat ghee in a large frying pan or wok over moderate heat. Add mustard seeds. When they begin to pop add the remaining spices. Stir-fry over low heat for 1 minute. Then add zucchini and increase heat to moderately high. Fry uncovered until just tender. Stir frequently. Add tomatoes and salt. Stir and cook for 3 or 4 minutes more. Serve with rice or pasta.

## Almond Custard Fresh Fruit Pie

A sweet, easily digested pie that is good for building muscles, bones, brain and body tissues as well as fat, this dessert reduces Vata and Pitta, rather than Kapha. When served warm, the filling alone makes a nourishing custard for children.

Makes one 10-inch deep dish pie or tart

For the Butter Crust:

> 1 3/4 cups flour
> 1/4 teaspoon salt
> 1/2 cup butter
> 2 to 3 tablespoons cold water

Preheat oven to 425°

Mix dry ingredients. Cut in butter until just mealy looking. Sprinkle two tablespoons water over the mixture and blend lightly with a fork. Add remaining water as needed to make the dough form a ball. Roll gently between wax paper or a pastry cloth. Place in pie pan or tart shell, flute, prick with a fork, and bake for 12 to 15 minutes. Cool.

For the Filling:

> 1/4 cup cornstarch
> 1/2 cup sugar
> 2 cups half and half
> 2 cups whipping cream
> 1 1/2 cups ground blanched almonds
> 2 teaspoons almond extract
> 1 1/2 cups fresh fruit, such as whole or sliced strawberries, raspberries, or sliced kiwi and apricots

In a heavy 2-quart pan mix cornstarch and sugar. Cook over moderate heat, slowly stirring in the creams. Stir constantly and when just beginning to thicken add almonds. Lower to simmer and cook, stirring until just boiling and thick. Remove from heat and stir in almond extract. Pour into pie shell. Refrigerate until ready to serve. Decorate with fruit just before serving.

## American Apple Pie

This is a pleasantly spicy pie that is sweet and heavy. It decreases Vata and Pitta, and increases Kapha. By reducing the sugar and eliminating the nutmeg, Kapha can eat some of this pie. Or follow the Apple Pie without Sugar recipe.

Pie crust for top and bottom of 9-inch pie

    3 to 4 cups apples—peeled, cored, and chopped
    1/2 cup sugar
    4 tablespoons brown sugar
    1 1/2 teaspoons cinnamon
    3/4 teaspoon cardamom
    1/4 teaspoon nutmeg
    Juice of one lemon

Preheat oven to 375°.

Mix all ingredients in a large bowl. Roll out half the pie crust dough on a floured surface. Carefully place it in a 9-inch pan without tearing. Heap apples toward the center of the pan. Roll out the rest of the dough and lay it on the apples. Seal the edges well and slit vents in the top to allow steam to escape. Bake on a cookie sheet for about one hour or until crust is nicely browned.

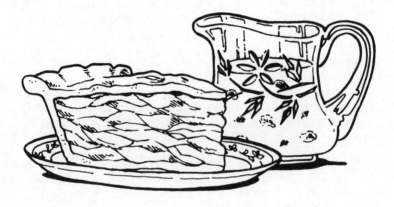

## Apple Dumplings with Vanilla Sauce

Everyone loves apple dumplings. They are sweet and heavy, good for Vata and Pitta and increasing for Kapha. (Kapha can have a small dumpling without the sauce). This recipe's been tried and tested by many generations of Rick Weller's family. Because it doesn't get soggy the Rich Dumpling Crust, when the ingredients are doubled, makes an excellent pastry for cream and fruit pies.

Serves 4 to 5

Rich Dumpling Crust:
3/4 cups butter or shortening
1 1/2 cups unbleached flour
1/2 teaspoon salt
1 teaspoon plain yogurt
1 1/2 teaspoons white vinegar
2 1/2 tablespoons cold water

Cut butter into flour and salt. Mix yogurt, vinegar, and water together, then add to the dough. Form into a ball, cover, and chill while preparing the apples.

4 to 5 baking apples
1/2 cup brown sugar
1 teaspoon cinnamon
4 to 5 tablespoons butter
Preheat oven to 425°.

Peel and core the apples. In a small bowl mix brown sugar and cinnamon together. On a floured surface roll out dough thin. Cut it into 4 or 5 equal squares. Place an apple in the center of each square, fill each cored apple with a tablespoon of brown sugar mixture, and top with a tablespoon of butter. Wrap the pastry over the apple, sealing well. Use a little milk or water to seal the edges closed. Place on baking sheet that has sides and bake for 10 minutes. Reduce heat to 350° for 30 more minutes or until nicely brown. Serve warm with Vanilla Sauce.

## Vanilla Sauce

When served warm in a pitcher or small gravy boat Vanilla Sauce makes something special of fruit dumplings, unfrosted cakes, waffles, pancakes, and apple pie . It decreases Vata and Pitta, and increases Kapha.

Makes 2 1/2 cups

3/4 cups sugar
2 tablespoons cornstarch
1/4 teaspoon salt
2 cups boiling water
1/4 cup raisins or currants (optional)
1 tablespoon vanilla
4 tablespoons butter
Dash nutmeg

Mix dry ingredients in a heavy saucepan. Add boiling water and raisins. Stir constantly over moderate heat until the sauce shimmers and looks clear and thickened, about 5 minutes. Remove from heat and stir in vanilla, butter, and nutmeg. Continue stirring until butter is melted. Serve warm. Refrigerate and reheat as needed. This sauce keeps for two or three days covered in refrigerator.

## Apple Pie Filling without Sugar

For those watching their weight but still wishing eat a good slice of American apple pie or a turnover, this is the filling to choose. A flour crust will add to its Kapha-increasing properties, but not very much. It reduces Vata and Pitta.

Pie crust for top and bottom of 9-inch pie

10 medium baking apples—Granny Smith, Jonathan, or Winesap
Juice of one large lemon or two medium oranges
3/4 cup raisins
3 tablespoons cornstarch
2 tablespoons cinnamon

Preheat oven to 425°.

Peel and slice apples very thinly. Add remaining ingredients and mix thoroughly. Roll out half the pie crust dough on a floured surface. Carefully place it in a 9-inch pan without tearing. Heap apples toward the center of the pan. Roll out the rest of the dough and lay it on the apples. Seal the edges well and cut slits in the top. Bake on a cookie sheet for 15 minutes at 425° then reduce to 350° and bake 45 minutes longer.

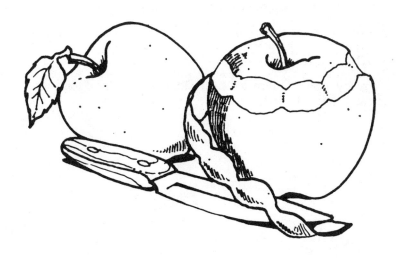

## Chocolate Custard Pie

This delicious, sweet, unctuous (oily), astringent, bitter pie filling decreases Vata and Pitta and increases Kapha. It is good for increasing weight.

9-inch Pre-baked pie crust

1 pint half and half cream
1 pint whipping cream
1/4 cup cornstarch
1/2 cup sugar
1/2 teaspoon vanilla
6 oz. semi-sweet chocolate chips
1/4 cup chocolate chips
1 cup sweetened whipped cream
Shaved bitter chocolate, optional

In a small bowl mix cornstarch and sugar together and set aside. Heat creams over low heat or in the top of a double boiler. Add small amount of steamy cream to the dry ingredients and whisk to blend. When smooth pour slowly into the rest of the cream whisking all the time. Stir constantly until thickened. Remove from heat and add vanilla and chocolate chips. Stir until blended. Cover with plastic wrap directly on filling and refrigerate until cold.

Meanwhile bake pie shell. When it comes out of the oven spread chocolate chips evenly on the bottom and let cool. If chips do not melt entirely slip the pan back in the turned off oven for a minute or two.

When ready to serve, fill cooled shell with the custard and top with whipped cream and chocolate shavings.

## Strawberry Yogurt Pie

This makes a pretty pie that is not too filling to eat after a big meal. It's sour, sweet, cold, oily, and heavy properties decrease Vata, are neutral for Pitta, and increase Kapha. It is a good pie to serve as a luncheon dessert or in the afternoon with tea. Because of the sour yogurt, it should not be eaten too late at night.

1 pre-baked 9-inch pie shell, cooled

4-ounce packaged cream cheese
8-ounce. container strawberry yogurt
8-ounces. kefir cheese or ricotta cheese
4 tablespoons sugar
1 cup sliced strawberries
10-12 whole strawberries, or more to taste, washed and stemmed

Blend cheeses together. Add yogurt and sugar. Blend well. Refrigerate until solid. Spread sliced fruit on bottom of baked pie crust and cover with yogurt mixture. Refrigerate until ready to serve and top with more sliced fruit before serving.

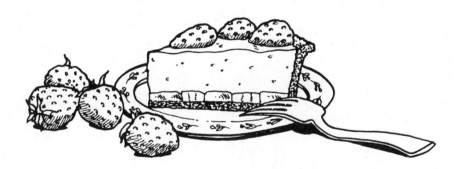

## Swedish Chocolate Cream Pie

A luscious, richly creamy pie made sweeter and more unctuous with white chocolate, this is a real winner for Vata and Pitta. It is a quick, no-bake pie that uses any sweet, seasonally available fruits to advantage.

Makes one 10-inch pie

Prebake 10-inch pie crust

2 1/2 tablespoons cornstarch or arrowroot
2 cups milk
3 tablespoons sugar
4 ounces white chocolate, broken in pieces
1 teaspoon vanilla
8 ounces sour cream
2 cups berries, sliced peaches, or other sweet fruit
1 cup stiffly whipped cream

In a heavy sauce pan mix cornstarch and 1/3 cup milk. Add remaining milk and stir over moderately low flame until at boiling point. Stir vigorously for 5 minutes to cook cornstarch. Add white chocolate and continue stirring for 5 more minutes. Remove from heat and beat in vanilla and sour cream. Turn into pie pan and freeze for 30 minutes, if in a hurry or chill in refrigerator for two hours. Then decorate with whole or sliced fruit, pipe on whipped cream, and refrigerate another hour or until ready to serve.

## Sweet Potato-Apple Pie

This is a sweet, heavy dessert for Vata and Pitta diets. When made without the pie crust it's a good side dish to a main meal.

Makes an 8-inch pie

1 unbaked 8-inch single pie crust

1 large sweet potato, baked
1 sweet apple, peeled and shredded
1/8 cup sweet orange, pineapple, or apple juice
1/4 cup brown sugar
1/4 cup blanched almonds, finely ground
  or
  1/4 cup coconut
1/4 teaspoon cinnamon
1/8 teaspoon ginger and nutmeg mixed

Preheat oven to 350°.

Peel potato and mash with other ingredients. Spread on pie crust. Bake for 30 to 40 minutes or until crust is nicely browned and tines of fork in center come out clean. Cool at least 10 minutes before cutting.

## Butter Crust

All pie crusts in this book are made from wheat flour. They decrease Vata and Pitta and increase Kapha.

Makes two 10-inch crusts

3 cups flour
1/4 teaspoon salt
1 cup cold butter
3 to 4 tablespoons ice water

Mix flour and salt together, then cut in butter with a pastry cutter, or chop with a knife until pieces are the size of currants or small peas. Add the ice water a tablespoon at a time, just until the dough will hold together to form a ball. Roll out on a floured surface. Try not to stretch or handle the dough more than necessary or it will become tough.

## Oil Pastry

This flaky crust can be made quickly in a food processor using the steel blade. Also by stirring with a fork.

Makes two 9-inch crusts

2 cups flour
1 teaspoon salt
1/2 cup oil
4 to 5 tablespoons cold water

In a processor bowl mix flour and salt. In a separate cup, first pour the oil, then 4 tablespoons water, but do not mix. Pour them slowly into the processor while it is running. It should make a soft dough. Add a little more water, if necessary. Roll out on a floured surface, or press right into the bottom of the pie pan.

Halve recipe for a single, filled pie. Prick with fork and bake 12 minutes before filling.

## Simple Cookie Crust

This basic unbaked crust can be used for all cream pies. Sweet and oily, it increases Kapha, but is good for Pitta and Vata.

Makes two 8-inch crusts or one 10-inch.

2 cups graham cracker or other cookie crumbs
1/2 cup ghee or butter
4 tablespoons sugar

Preheat oven to 400°.

Mix all ingredients in a food processor with a steel blade or in a large bowl. Press the mixture into a pie pan and bake for 5 to 8 minutes, until just tan colored. Cool and fill.

## Cashew Nut Balls or Squares

Cashew Nut Balls, also known as Laddus (LAh-dooz), are ball-shaped, un-baked sweets like a cookie and candy combined. If not made in balls, the dough can be pressed into a 9-inch square pan, dusted with confectioner's sugar, and cut into 1-inch squares when hardened. This sweet, unctuous, and slightly heavy dessert is good for Vata and Pitta, and in small amounts good for Kapha, too.

Makes 1 1/2 dozen

1 teaspoon ghee
3 tablespoons cashews
4 tablespoons ghee
1 cup besan (chickpea) flour, from Asian or natural food store, or substitute whole wheat flour
6 green cardamom pods, seeded and ground
          or
   1/2 teaspoon fresh ground cardamom
1 cup brown sugar

Melt 1 teaspoon ghee in a small pan over low heat. Add nuts and fry until lightly toasted. Remove from heat and chop fine in nut grinder. Set aside.

In a large skillet or heavy pan heat 4 tablespoons ghee. Add besan and cook over low heat, stirring frequently until golden. Watch carefully not to allow the flour to get too dark. Remove from heat and add the nuts and other ingredients, stirring well. The dough will leave the sides of the pan and be thick when well mixed. Cool until it can be handled, about 30 minutes. Roll each laddu into a small ball, smaller than a golf ball. Rub hands with ghee if dough sticks too much.

Arrange on a plate as they are rolled and set aside at least an hour, or until they are hard, before serving. Store in a tightly sealed container.

## Fresh Ginger Cookies

Here is a cookie that is easy to make *and* good for all doshas.   It's one of those rare desserts that Kapha can eat in more than in small amounts.  These cookies reduce Kapha and Vata, and have a neutral effect on Pitta.  They are sweet, pungent, salty, and astringent. Made entirely with barley flour, one of Kapha's best grains, and include a generous amount of ginger, they actually benefit weight watchers.  Using fresh ginger really makes these sparkle!

These cookies travel well for sending as gifts.

Makes about 2 dozen

> 4 cups barley flour
> 2 teaspoons baking soda
> 1/4 teaspoon salt
> 1 tablespoon cinnamon
> 1/2 teaspoon cloves
> 1/2 cup oil or ghee
> 1 1/3 cups molasses
> 3 tablespoons fresh ginger, finely grated
>              or
>   1 tablespoon ground ginger

Preheat oven to 350°.

Mix all ingredients together and roll into 1-inch balls. Bake on a lightly greased cookie sheet for about 15 minutes or until light brown.  The centers will be soft. Cool on a rack and store securely.

## Italian Hazelnut Cookies

These delicate cookies are sweet, bitter, astringent, dry, and good for all doshas. When made with both wheat and barley flour they are best for Kapha. If you don't have barley flour on hand, use all white flour. These cookies pack well to send as gifts. The anise flavor develops best when they are stored in a sealed container for a day or two.

Makes 2 1/2 dozen

   1 cup butter (1/2 pound), softened at room temperature
   1/4 cup sugar
   2 teaspoons anise extract
            or
      3 teaspoons ground anise seeds
   1/2 cup barley flour
   1 1/2 cups unbleached white flour
            or
      2 cups unbleached white flour
   1/4 teaspoon salt
   3/4 cup finely ground hazelnuts (or pecans)
   1/2 cup powdered sugar

Preheat oven to 300°.

Cream butter and sugar together. Mix in anise extract or ground seeds. Measure dry ingredients in a separate bowl and mix together thoroughly. Stir in nuts, then add dry ingredients to the butter mixture.

Shape into balls or 2 x2 1/2-inch crescents. Roll in powdered sugar. Bake on ungreased cookie sheets in the center of the oven until faintly brown, about 12 minutes. (Gently turn one cookie over to test for color.) When cool roll again in powdered sugar.

## Jam Diagonals

A fancy and easily made bar cookie that is a fine treat for Vata and Pitta, it adds sweet, heavy aspects to a meal.

Makes about 2 dozen cookies

    1/4 cup granulated sugar
    1/2 cup softened butter
    1 teaspoon vanilla
    1/8 teaspoon salt
    1 1/4 cups flour
    1/2 cup strawberry or raspberry jam
    3/4 cup powdered sugar
    4 teaspoons lemon juice

Preheat oven to 350°.

For the dough:

Beat sugar, butter, vanilla, and salt together in a mixing bowl until fluffy. Stir in flour and blend well. Divide dough in thirds. Using hands roll each third into a 9-inch rope. Place 3 inches apart on ungreased cookie sheet. With finger make 1/2-inch depression down the center of each rope. The ropes will flatten to 1-inch wide strips.

Fill the depressions with jam. Bake for 12 to 15 minutes until golden. Cool on the sheet.

For the Icing:

In a small bowl blend powdered sugar and lemon juice until smooth; then drizzle over the jam. When icing is set, cut diagonally in one-inch bars.

## Lemony Date Bars

These bar cookies are not only sweet and delicious, but are good for you, too. The fruit and grain combinations are especially nourishing for Vata and Pitta, but increase Kapha by building muscles and tissues. Because the are so nutritious everyone can eat them in moderation. When cut in 3-inch squares and served in small bowls with heavy cream poured over the top they make a fine dessert for Vata and Pitta.

Makes 1 1/2 dozen

　　2 cups pitted dates, chopped
　　2/3 cup white sugar
　　1 cup water
　　1/4 cup lemon peel, coarsely chopped
　　Juice of 1/2 lemon
　　1 cup white flour
　　1 cup whole wheat flour
　　2 cups brown sugar, packed
　　1 teaspoon salt
　　1 cup ( 1/2 pound) butter or margarine
　　3 cups oats
　　1/3 cup milk
　　2 teaspoons vanilla

Preheat oven to 350°.

In a heavy saucepan cook dates, white sugar, and water until thick and well blended. Add lemon peel and lemon juice to date mixture. Stir well and cool. Mix flour, brown sugar, and salt together in a large bowl. Cut in shortening until well blended. A food processor with a large bowl is good for this job. Add oatmeal and mix well. Mix milk and vanilla together then blend into dough. Pack a thin layer of dough on the bottom of a greased 13-inch by 9-inch pan or two 8-inch by 8-inch pans. Spread fruit on top and pat remaining dough over fruit. The dough does not have to cover the fruit completely. It will spread during baking. Bake 30 to 40 minutes until brown on top. Cool, cut into bars.

## Mother's Laddu

These sweet, unctuous (oily) cookies are both nourishing and satisfying. They come from the new mother's recipes, but anyone can eat them especially those following a regular Vata or Pitta-reducing diet. Kapha could have one or two. If there is not enough time to roll them into balls, just pat the dough into an 8-inch square pan and allow to set until firm, then cut into 1-inch squares. Cashew Nut Balls recipe is a variation on this one.

Makes about 1 1/2 dozen

    4 tablespoon ghee
    3 tablespoons blanched almonds, finely ground
    1 cup besan (chickpea flour from an Asian or natural food store)
    6 green cardamom pods, seeded and ground
            or
      1/2 teaspoon fresh ground cardamom
    1 cup brown sugar

In a large skillet or heavy pan heat 4 tablespoons ghee. Add ground almonds and besan flour. Cook over low heat, stirring frequently until golden. Watch closely not to allow the flour to get too dark. Remove from heat and add the other ingredients, stirring well. The dough will leave the sides of the pan and be thick when it is well mixed.

Cool just until it can be handled, about 30 minutes. Roll each laddu into a small ball, smaller than a golf ball. Rub hands with ghee if the dough sticks too much.

Arrange them on a plate as they are rolled and set aside for at least an hour, or until they are hard, then serve. Store in a tightly sealed container.

## Oatmeal Raisin Cookies

Highly nutritious and tasty, these cookies ship well and are very good for dunking. Both Vata and Pitta can eat these sweet, heavy, slightly salty cookies. They increase Kapha, but are so nutritious that Kapha can occasionally have a couple.

Makes 4 to 5 dozen

1/3 cup oil
1/2 cup margarine or butter
1 cup white sugar
1 cup brown sugar, packed
1/3 cup milk
2 teaspoons vanilla
1 1/2 cups white flour
1 cup whole wheat flour
1 teaspoon baking powder
1 teaspoon baking soda
1 teaspoon salt
3 cups oats
1 cup raisins
1/2 cup walnuts, broken

Preheat oven to 350°.

Cream margarine and oil. Then add sugars and cream well. Add milk and vanilla. In a separate bowl mix together flour, baking soda, baking powder, and salt. Stir into sugar mixture. Add oats, raisins, and nuts. Mix with fingers if it's too thick to stir. Shape into balls and flatten slightly. Place close together, but not touching, on greased baking sheets. Bake 15 minutes until just turning brown underneath.

## Simple Shortbread

A rich unleavened dessert for everyone, shortbread can be served more festively with jam spread on top.

Makes 1 dozen


    1/2 pound (2 sticks) butter
    1/2 cup sugar—or more to taste
    2 cups unbleached flour
    1/4 teaspoon salt

Preheat oven to 350°.

Cream butter thoroughly with the sugar. Mix flour and salt together, then add to the butter mixture. Roll or pat out dough to a 1/4-inch thickness, cut into 1-inch by 2-inch rectangles, and prick several times with a fork. Place with sides not touching on an ungreased baking sheet. Bake 20 to 25 minutes or until light brown on edges.


**Faster Method:** Pat dough into a 9-inch pie pan, prick all over the top, and bake 25 to 30 minutes. Cut when warm.

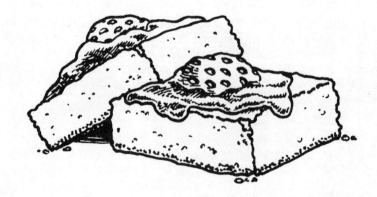

## Super Chocolate Brownies

This is a rich chocolate brownie that is good for anyone who likes chocolate. The tastes are bitter, sweet, astringent, a little salty, and very delicious. The only thing wrong with these brownies is that you have to wait until they are completely cool to cut them. They are best made by hand and not with an electric mixer.

Makes 1 dozen brownies

1/2 cup butter or ghee
2 squares (2 ounces) unsweetened chocolate
1/3 cup flour
1 1/4 cups cool water
1/2 teaspoon salt
2 teaspoons vanilla
1/2 cup cocoa (best quality available)
2 cups flour
2 teaspoons baking powder
2 cups sugar
1 cup pecans or blanched almonds, coarsely chopped

Grease a 9 x 12-inch pan. Preheat oven to 350°.

For the Chocolate Mixture:

Stir and melt the chocolate squares and butter together in a small heavy pan over low heat. Set aside when well-blended. In a small saucepan mix 1/3 cup flour with a little water to make a paste, then add the remaining water and cook over moderate heat, stirring constantly, until thickened, about 5 minutes. A few lumps are okay. Remove from heat and stir in salt, vanilla, and chocolate mixture.

To Combine:

Measure dry ingredients into a large bowl. Stir well or sift together. Mix in sugar, liquid mixture, and then the nuts. Stir until just blended, about one minute. The mixture will look very thick. Spread into the pan and bake for 25 to 30 minutes on the center oven rack. Brownies are done when they just start to leave the edges of the pan. For moist brownies, a knife inserted in the middle will not come out completely clean. Remove from the oven and cool completely before cutting.

## Toasty Cinnamon Bar Cookies

Good for Vata, Pitta, and increases Kapha and these cookies are simple to make. They just seem to "disappear" as soon as they are cut into bars.

Makes 1 1/2 dozen

For the Batter:

>  2 cups flour
>  1 cup sugar
>  1/2 teaspoon salt
>  2 teaspoons baking powder
>  1 cup milk
>  1 tablespoon ghee or melted butter
>  1 teaspoon vanilla
>  1/2 cup raisins
>  1/2 cup pecans, chopped

Preheat oven to 350°.

Combine all ingredients. Spread in 15 x 10 inch sheet pan. Bake 20 minutes. While bars bake, mix the topping.

For the Topping:

>  1/2 cup ghee or melted butter
>  1/2 cup sugar
>  1 1/2 teaspoons cinnamon

Drizzle over baked cookie dough, spreading evenly. Bake 10 more minutes. Cool and cut into bars.

## Fruit Shortcake

A favorite American dessert, shortcake is quick to make and good for Vata and Pitta. With sweet, astringent, slightly salty tastes, and heavy, dry qualities, the cake alone is good for all doshas. But the addition of whipped cream and sweet fruit increases the sweet, cold, and heavy qualities. Since these increase Kapha, moderation is necessary. This is not a dessert for weight watchers.

Sweet fruits like berries, sweet cherries, and ripe peaches are the best choices to serve with whipped cream. For strawberry shortcake select only the sweetest variety and lightly sprinkle them with sugar before using.

For the Cake:

> 1/2 cup besan (chickpea) or barley flour
> 2 cups unbleached white flour
> 2 teaspoons baking powder
> 1/4 cup sugar
> 1/2 teaspoon salt
> 4 tablespoons unsalted butter or ghee
> 1/2 cup milk

Grease an 8-inch pan. Preheat oven to 450°.

In a large bowl sift or stir the dry ingredients together. Rub the butter in with your fingers. Add enough milk to make a soft dough. Pat into baking pan and bake for 15 to 20 minutes until slightly brown on top. Cool and remove from pan.

Before Serving:

> 4 cups fresh fruit, peeled and cut in bite-size pieces
> 1/2 cup sugar
> 1 cup whipping cream
> 1 teaspoon vanilla extract

Sprinkle fruit with sugar (less than 1 tablespoon) and set aside for at least 20 minutes. Whip cream and add the reserved sugar and vanilla. Serve on sliced shortcake.

## Ginger Spice Cake with Lemon Sauce

A simple cake to make for Vata and Kapha. Pitta would have just a little less of this pungent and sweet unfrosted cake. It's especially nice to serve on a cold afternoon in winter.

Makes an 8-inch square cake

        1 1/2 cup unbleached flour, sifted
        1/2 cup sugar
        3/4 teaspoon baking powder
        3/4 teaspoon baking soda
        1/2 teaspoon salt
        2 teaspoons fresh ginger, grated
                    or
          1 teaspoon ground ginger
        1 teaspoon cinnamon
        1/4 teaspoon allspice
        1/4 teaspoon nutmeg
        1/4 cup corn syrup
        1/4 cup warm ghee or melted butter
        1/2 cup buttermilk or sour raw milk
        3 tablespoons plain yogurt
        1/2 cup water

Grease 8-inch square pan. Preheat oven to 350°.

Mix dry ingredients and spices together. In a separate bowl thoroughly blend syrup, ghee, buttermilk, and yogurt. Add to dry ingredients and beat for 2 minutes. Then add enough water to make a thick but pourable batter. Pour into pan and bake. Allow to cool before cutting. Serve with a small pitcherful of Lemon Sauce.

## Lemon Sauce

A refreshing topping for plain and spicy cakes that is good for Vata, this sauce increases Pitta and Kapha somewhat.

Makes about 1 cup

    3/4 cup sugar
    1 tablespoon plus 2 teaspoons cornstarch
    pinch of salt
    1/2 cup boiling water
    1 teaspoon grated lemon peel
    3 tablespoons lemon juice (one half of a squeezed lemon)
    3 tablespoons butter

In a small saucepan mix sugar, cornstarch, and salt. Whisk in boiling water and simmer ten minutes over moderate heat. Add remaining ingredients stir over low heat until the butter melts. Serve warm.

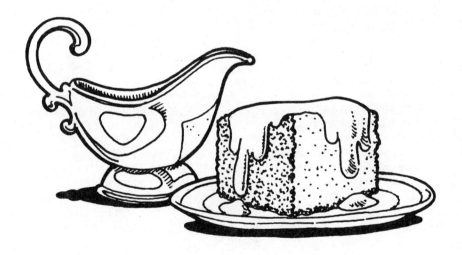

## Marble Crumb Cake with Vanilla Sauce and English Cream

This heavenly cake, simply made by layering a crumb cake mixture with sweet syrup and then tracing swirls in the batter with a knife to marble, is served with a pitcher of warm Vanilla Sauce and unsweetened heavy cream whipped with cream cheese. It is sweet, oily, slightly sour, good for Vata with neutral effects for Pitta. Kapha would eat this cake without the sauce and whipped cream.

Serves 4 to 6

> 2 1/2 cup unbleached flour
> 1 teaspoon baking powder
> Dash salt
> 1/4 cup white sugar
> 3/4 cups brown sugar, firmly packed
> 3/4 cup butter
> 1/2 cup corn syrup
> 1/2 cup light molasses
> 1 teaspoon baking soda
> 1 cup boiling water

Grease 8 x 8 x 2-inch baking pan. Preheat oven to 375°.

Measure flour into a mixing bowl, or in food processor using steel blade. Add baking powder, salt, white sugar, and brown sugar. Blend well. Cut in butter until it resembles coarse crumbs. In a small bowl combine syrup, molasses, baking soda, and boiling water.

Press 1 cup of crumb mixture firmly into bottom of baking pan. Pour in 2/3 cup syrup mixture. Spread another crumb layer on top, followed by syrup. Make three layers in all. Sprinkle remaining crumb mixture on top. Using a knife or spatula, gently cut through batter in swirling motions to marble. Avoid cutting through the bottom pressed crumb layer. Bake in center of oven for about 45 minutes until firm and brown and a cake tester comes out clean. Cool on a rack.

When ready to serve cut into squares, pour on generous amounts of Vanilla Sauce, and top with a dollop of English cream.

## Vanilla Sauce

Serve warm in a pitcher or small gravy boat over unfrosted cakes, waffles, pancakes, fruit dumplings, and apple pie. It decreases Vata and Pitta, and increases Kapha.

Makes 2 1/2 cups

    3/4 cup sugar
    2 tablespoons cornstarch
    1/4 teaspoon salt
    2 cups boiling water
    1/4 cup raisins or currants (optional)
    1 tablespoon vanilla
    4 tablespoons butter
    Dash nutmeg

Mix dry ingredients in a heavy saucepan. Add boiling water and raisins. Stir constantly over moderate heat until the sauce shimmers and looks clear and thickened, about 5 minutes. Remove from heat and stir in vanilla, butter, and nutmeg. Continue stirring until butter is melted. Serve warm. Refrigerate and reheat as needed. This sauce keeps for two or three days covered in refrigerator.

## English Cream

As a garnish for cakes and scones this sweet, sour, cold, heavy cream is better for Vata than Pitta or Kapha.

    3 tablespoons cream cheese
    1/2 pint heavy cream
    1/4 teaspoon vanilla

Whip until soft and fluffy.

## Old Fashioned Tea Cake

A wonderfully rich, orange-flavored, moist old-fashioned cake, its sweet, nourishing, heavy, and oily properties arebest for Vata and Pitta. Dates add to the elegant heaviness, but currants or raisins work equally well.

    1 cup chopped dates, raisins, or currants
    Zest of 3 oranges, minced
    1 cup sugar
    1/2 cup butter
    6 tablespoons yogurt
    3/4 cup whole milk (or buttermilk)
    1 teaspoon vanilla
    2 cups unbleached flour
    2 teaspoons baking soda
    2 teaspoons baking powder
    1/2 teaspoon salt
    1/2 cup walnuts, finely ground
    2 tablespoons water

Grease 9-inch tube pan.  Preheat oven to 325°.

In food processor or blender grind orange peel and dates together until fine. Cream sugar and butter together.  Add yogurt, milk, and vanilla and mix thoroughly.  Mix dry ingredients separately and stir into butter mixture.  Mix nuts and water together and fold into batter.  Pour into tube pan.  Bake until cake tests done by inserting toothpick or wooden skewer into center, about 50 to 55 minutes.  Do not open oven before 50 minutes  to check.  This is one of those cakes that collapses if bothered too early.  Remove from oven and let stand in pan for 10 minutes before removing.

While cake is baking mix orange marinade:

    1 cup fresh orange juice
    1/2 cup sugar
    2 teaspoons vanilla

In a small pan heat and stir ingredients over moderate flame until sugar is dissolved.  Then slowly pour over the cake a tablespoon at a time.  Cover cake and and set aside until completely cool.  Serve with softly whipped cream.

## Sweet Chocolate Cake With Cherry Sauce

Like an elegant Black Forest Cake but easier to make, this dessert is sweet, slightly bitter, oily, and heavy. It reduces Vata and Pitta, and increases Kapha. The tofu and banana make it especially nourishing for body tissues. It can be made as an elaborate layer cake with a rich chocolate mousse filling, or simply in one layer topped with warm dark cherry sauce.

Makes one 8-inch layer cake or a single sheet cake

For the Cake:

> 1/2  cup (1 stick) butter
> 3 ounces sweet chocolate
> 2 cups unbleached flour
> 1 cup sugar
> 1/3 cup cocoa (best quality)
> 1 teaspoon baking powder
> 1 teaspoon baking soda
> 1/4 teaspoon salt
> 1/2 pound tofu
> 1 small ripe banana
> 1/2 cup milk
> 1/2 cup chopped nuts, (optional)

Preheat oven to 350°.

Grease and dust with flour two 8-inch pans or a 9 x13-inch sheet pan.

Melt butter and chocolate in a small pan over low heat. Stir until blended. then set aside while preparing other ingredients.

In a large bowl stir dry ingredients together. Blend the tofu, milk, and banana in a food processor or with an electric mixer until thick and creamy. Combine all ingredients, pour into pans, and bake for 30 minutes or until a knife inserted in the middle comes out clean. Allow pans to rest for 5 to 10 minutes before removing cakes. Cool before filling.

The single layer sheet cake can be cut and served with warm cherry sauce and whipped cream. Or prepare the layer cake as follows.

continues

## Sweet Chocolate Cake With Cherry Sauce,  continued

For the Cherry Sauce:

> 1 package (16 ounces) frozen dark, sweet cherries, defrosted
> 2 tablespoons sugar
> 1 tablespoon cornstarch
> 1 tablespoon cool water
> 1/2 teaspoon almond extract

Heat the cherries in a saucepan over moderate heat. Add the sugar and stir until dissolved. Turn to low and mix the cornstarch with water in a cup, then stir into the cherries. Return to moderate heat and continue stirring for about one minute until thickened. Remove from heat and add almond extract. Cool ten minutes before using.

Makes 2 cups

To Assemble Layer Cake:

Spread 1 1/2 cups chocolate mousse filling out to half an inch from the edge of the bottom layer. Gently place second layer on top (this cake is very tender to handle), then spread warm cherry sauce on top, allowing it to drizzle over the sides. Garnish with piped remaining mousse or whipped cream and shaved bitter chocolate.

## Sweet Fruit and Spice Tea Bread

The particular combination of fruits and spices in this sweet bread gives it all the qualities of a good rasayana—something that is fundamentally nourishing for everyone at the start of digestion. Preparation time is longer than for many desserts, but this one is worth it. It is a sweet, astringent, slightly bitter dessert bread that is good for balancing all doshas. Although the ghee and butter increase weight a bit, this delicious bread is very good for Vata and Pitta, and nourishing for Kapha when eaten moderately.

Makes one large loaf

For the Dough:

    2 tablespoons dry yeast—"rapid rise" works best
    1 1/2 cups apple juice, heated
    1/2 cup warm water
    14 cup sugar
    1/4 cup ghee or melted butter
    1 teaspoon lemon peel
    1/2 teaspoon cinnamon
    1/2 teaspoon allspice
    1/2 teaspoon nutmeg
    1/4 teaspoon cloves
    1 teaspoon salt
    2 cups whole wheat flour
    3 to 4 cups unbleached white flour

For the Filling:

    1/2 cup dried apricots
    1/2 cup dried peaches
    1/2 cup pitted prunes
    1 cup boiling water
    1 1/2 cup blanched almonds, chopped
    3/4 cup poppy seeds
    1/2 cup butter
    1/2 cup brown sugar, packed
    2 teaspoons cinnamon

continues

## Sweet Fruit and Spice Tea Bread continued

For the Icing:

    1 tablespoon orange juice
    3 tablespoons powdered sugar

Make the filling :

Chop dried fruit and place in a 1-quart bowl. Pour enough boiling water over the fruit to cover. Cover and let stand for 4 or 5 hours or overnight. Soak until very soft. When ready to mix, measure 2 cups softened, drained fruit with remaining ingredients. Stir well. Set aside while making the sweet dough.

Preheat oven to 350°.

Make the Dough:

In a large bowl blend yeast, sugar, warm juice, and water. Let this sit for 5 to 10 minutes until frothy. Add ghee, lemon peel, spices, salt, and whole wheat flour. Blend everything together and then stir vigorously for 2 minutes. Stir in white flour a cup at a time until a stiff dough is formed.

Turn out on a floured board and knead until smooth and not sticky, about 10 minutes. Wash bowl and rub with a little ghee. Put dough in the bowl, spread a little ghee on top to keep it moist, and cover with plastic wrap or a clean towel. Let rise in a warm place until double in bulk, about 1 hour. Punch down, cover, and let it rise again until double in bulk, another hour.

Punch down and turn out on lightly floured board. Roll into a long rectangle with a rolling pin. The size will be about 16 x 10 inches. Stir filling again and spread evenly over dough. Roll tightly beginning at the long end. Pinch ends together to close. Place on a greased baking sheet, cover, and let rise about an hour or until evenly puffy.

Bake bread 25 to 35 minutes until it is golden brown on top and sounds a little hollow when tapped on the bottom. Cool on a rack.

Mix orange juice and powdered sugar together to make icing. Dribble over top of the top.

# Creamy Rice Pudding

This rich, nourishing dessert is sweet, heavy, and slightly pungent. Rice pudding and other milk-based puddings are best for digestion when served warm. Long, slow cooking over low heat allows the rice grains to blend so well with the other ingredients that it becomes a creamy, easily digested treat.

Serves 4 to 6

    3 cups water
    2 cinnamon sticks
    1 cup long grain rice
    3 cups warm milk
    1 cup sugar
    1/2 cup raisins
    1/4 teaspoon crumbled saffron threads
    1/2 cup blanched almonds, finely chopped


Bring the water and cinnamon sticks to a boil in a large pot. Add the rice and simmer on low, covered, for about 15 to 20 minutes or until the water evaporates and the rice is soft. Meanwhile, mix the milk, sugar, raisins, saffron, and almonds in a bowl and set aside.

When the rice is soft, add the milk mixture to the pot and cook over moderately high heat until just boiling. Reduce heat to low and allow to simmer, uncovered, 20 to 30 minutes. Stir frequently. The pudding is done when everything is well blended and the rice grains can barely be seen. Pour into dishes and serve warm.

## Kaffa's Dream

A delightfully rich dessert that is sweet, heavy, oily, bitter, and slightly sour, this is the kind of chocolate pudding, cream-filled with crunchy crust confection, that you would serve at the conclusion of a very special dinner or as a party treat. Children love it. Eating some of Kaffa's Dream is good for Vata and has a neutral effect on Pitta. Eating any more than a bite should remain a "dream" for Kapha.

Makes 16 ramekins or one 13 x 9-inch pan

The crust:

> 2 1/4 cups graham cracker crumbs
> 1/2 cup unsalted butter, melted
> 1/2 cup sugar
> 1/2 to 3/4 cup flaked coconut
> 1/4 cup finely chopped pecans
> 1 (15-ounce) can sweetened condensed milk
> 8 ounces semi-sweet chocolate pieces

Combine all ingredients. Press two thirds of mixture into the pan or divide evenly among the 16 ramekins or custard cups. Reserve one third of mixture.

Preheat oven to 375°.

Heat milk in a saucepan over moderate heat. Blend in chocolate chips and stir until mixture thicken and chocolate is well blended. Pour over the crust, dividing equally among the cups. Sprinkle with remaining crumb mixture and press down. Bake for 12 minutes. Cool while preparing the two fillings.

The fillings:

> 8 ounces cream cheese, softened
> 1 cup powdered sugar
> 1/2 pint heavy cream, whipped
> 1 teaspoon vanilla
> 1/2 cup pecans, coarsely chopped

## Kaffa's Dream, continued

Beat cream cheese and sugar together in a small bowl. Fold in whipped cream and vanilla. Spread on top of the cooled chocolate crumb crust. Sprinkle with nuts. Refrigerate.

    1 large package (7 ounces) dark chocolate pudding
    ( or use the recipe for Chocolate Custard Pie Filling, if you have time)
    2 3/4 cups milk
    1/2 cup semi-sweet chocolate pieces

Mix the pudding with the milk following the package directions. Mix in the chocolate chips while pudding simmers. Let it cool and then pour over the chilled cream mixture. Chill for two or three hours.

Optional Finish:

In case this is not yet rich enough, top with great dollops of whipped cream, garnish with shaved bitter chocolate and a few fresh whole strawberries, raspberries, or other favorite fruit.

## Lemon Scones

Scones, a pleasant breakfast or teatime treat, are made like shortcake. Slivers of lemon peel, or orange peel if you prefer, add a delightful surprise. These scones are sweet, astringent, slightly salty, heavy, and dry. The astringent and dry aspects are good for Kapha. When eaten in moderation scones are good for all doshas.

Makes 1 dozen

2 cups unbleached flour
1/2 cup besan (chickpea) or barley flour
2 teaspoons baking powder
1/4 cup sugar
1/2 teaspooon salt
4 tablespoons butter
1 to 2 teaspoons coarsely chopped lemon peel
1/2 cup milk

Grease large baking sheet and preheat oven to 475°.

In a large bowl sift or stir the dry ingredients together. Cut butter in with a pastry cutter, or rub with your fingers until well combined. Add lemon peel and enough milk to make a soft dough. Roll out on floured board about 1/2 inch thick. With serrated knife or very sharp knife cut into triangles. Bake 10 to 12 minutes until lightly brown. Serve warm.

## Some substitutions for the lemon peel:

1/4 cup raisins or currants
2 large dates, chopped
2 teaspoons fresh or crystallized ginger, chopped
1/4 cup dried apricots, slivered

## Peche Cardinal

This is a combination of sweet tastes and heavy qualities good for both Vata and Pitta. Kapha types should eliminate the Chantilly cream and eat lightly of this dish.

Serves 6

> 4 cups water
> 1 1/2 cups sugar
> 6 large peaches, peeled, halved, and pitted
> 2 tablespoons vanilla

In a heavy saucepan bring water and sugar to a boil over high heat, stirring constantly until sugar dissolves. Boil 3 minutes, then reduce heat. Add peaches and vanilla. Simmer 15 minutes or until barely tender when tested with a fork. Cover and refrigerate while preparing other ingredients.

For the Cardinal Sauce:

> 2 10-ounce packages frozen raspberries, or 2 cups fresh raspberries, washed
> 2 tablespoons fine granulated or confectioners sugar

Drain raspberries in a sieve and purée with a wooden spoon. Discard seeds and pulp. Stir sugar into the raspberry juice and refrigerate in tightly covered container.

Cream Chantilly:

> 1/2 cup heavy cream, chilled
> 1 1/2 tablespoons sugar, fine granulated or confectioners
> 2 teaspoons vanilla

Whip cream until thick. Sprinkle in sugar and vanilla. Continue beating until it is firm enough to hold soft peaks.

To serve: Arrange peaches halves in individual dishes or on a platter. Spoon Cardinal Sauce over each peach. Top with Cream Chantilly. Use the leftover peach cooking syrup for poaching other fruit, if desired.

## Pineapple Ice

A perfect dessert for Pitta, especially on a hot day. Easy to make and so like authentic Italian ices that for Pitta, a bowl of Pineapple Ice is a fine way to end an Italian meal. Because it is so cold and sweet, Vata and Kapha should have much less of this dessert.

Makes 1 1/2 quarts

    1/4 -1/2 cup sugar, to taste
    2 cups water
    2 cups fresh pineapple, cored and chopped,
             or
      1 14-ounce can of crushed pineapple
    1/4 cup lemon juice

Boil the water and sugar in a heavy saucepan for 4 to 5 minutes, stirring until sugar is dissolved. Remove from heat, stir in pineapple and lemon juice. Cool and pour in a shallow bowl. Put in freezer. Every half hour remove and stir vigorously. When about half frozen whip with an electric mixer, on medium, for one minute. Freeze until firm.

## R&S Couscous

For those who want a warm filling start to the day, a quick, light evening meal, or something soothing on a day of light eating, prepare oatmeal, farina, rolled rye, or other cooked breakfast cereal with one or two teaspoons of ghee in the boiling water. Serve with warm milk or cream and sugar.

R & S (Rich and Satisfying) Couscous is a special Vata and Pitta-reducing cereal to serve for breakfast or a rather homey dessert.

Makes 2 1/2 cups

>   2 cups milk—or light cream for weight gaining
>   1 cup couscous
>   1 tablespoon ghee
>   1/4 to 1/2 cup raisins, currants, or chopped dates
>   Warm light cream or milk
>   Sugar to taste

Heat milk over moderate heat until just ready to boil. Add the couscous and and ghee. Stir vigorously with a wooden spoon until the liquid is almost absorbed. Stir in the fruit. When the cereal is steamy and begins to sizzle remove from heat. Cover and let sit for 5 to 10 minutes. Serve with warm cream or milk and sugar.

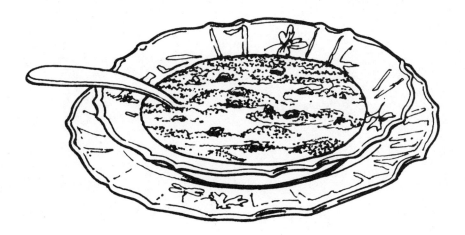

## Rich Quick Chocolate Mousse

This light chocolate mousse is useful either as a cake and pie filling, or served by itself at the end of an elegant dinner. With its sweet, bitter, oily, and heavy properties it is good for Pitta and Vata. Kapha would only have a small portion.

Makes 2 cups

2 cups heavy cream
4 ounces (1 bar) sweet baking chocolate
1 teaspoon vanilla

Heat cream in a heavy saucepan over low heat. When just simmering add chocolate in broken pieces. Stir until chocolate is melted and well blended. Cover and refrigerate 3 to 4 hours, or overnight. When ready to serve add vanilla and whip until stiff. Whipping this mixture will take less time than plain whipped cream does, about 2 minutes.

## To Make Mocha Mousse:

Add 2 tablespoons strong, cold coffee when ready to whip.

## White Figs a la Kapha

Although other figs like black or Mission figs are nourishing, none is held in such esteem by AyurVeda than Calmyrnas—known in sanskrit as *anjier*. Dried figs are sold at most supermarkets and natural food stores.

Plump some white Calmyrna figs in a vegetable steamer for 5 minutes. Serve warm. One or two figs and a few fresh ginger cookies make a good dessert for Kapha

## White Figs in Apricot Cream Sauce

Plain steamed figs are good for everyone who likes figs. This recipe makes a more elaborate dessert for Vata and Pitta,which can also be served at a breakfast/brunch or teatime party.

Serves 4

    10 to 12 Calmyrna figs
    1 1/2 cups heavy cream
    1/4 teaspoon nutmeg
    1/2 teaspoon cinnamon
    1 tablespoon apricot preserves
    fresh mint or lemon balm leaves, if available

Steam the figs for 5 minutes and set aside. When cool enough to handle slice each in half with a shape knife. Prepare the sauce.

In a heavy 2-quart saucepan heat the cream over a moderately high flame. Stir in the spices and preserves, whisking thoroughly. When cream just comes to a boil gently stir in the figs, coating them completely. Simmer over Serve immediately with mint or lemon balm leaf garnish.

# Chapter 11

# Questions and Answers about AyurVeda

# Questions and Answers about AyurVeda

by

Richard Averbach, M.D. and Dr. H. S. Kasture

1.     **Question:** What can everybody eat in winter or in summer?

**Answer:** Some of the dietary principles are really the same for all the prakritis—in cold, wet, or windy seasons heavier foods are best for everyone. In hot, humid seasons, lighter foods are best. From one point of view, it's not even the responsibility of the cook but your own responsibility to know what you should be eating. Because you are the one who actually chooses which foods to eat. So if you know that a certain type of food isn't so suitable for you at a particular time, then take less of that food.

2.     **Question:** Do the six tastes--sweet, sour, pungent, bitter, salty, and astringent--have to be in each dish in the meal? Can they be spread out in a whole meal, or taken over the whole day?

**Answer:** Each meal should have the six types of tastes. If you are taking two meals, one at lunch and one at dinner, both meals should have the six tastes. One dish may be sweet, another pungent or bitter, but all the dishes taken together should provide the full range. It is very difficult to include all six tastes in a single dish and have it be delicious.

3.     **Question:** Some children refuse to try all six tastes. How can we encourage them to eat something other than bread, milk, and pickles?

**Answer:** One has to prepare the meal according to the preferences of the children. That means six tastes should be mixed during the preparation into the food they like to eat. So make the foods they like best and mix in the six tastes. Eating habits can be changed gradually.

4.    **Question:** I'm Vata prakriti, my husband and children are other prakritis. How am I going to feed my whole family?

**Answer:** Balance is the theme of the entire dietary regimen. The principle of eating all six tastes and qualities at every meal will ensure a balanced diet for each family member. You can prepare balanced meals by following the guidelines in this book. Allow slight variations for different members of the family, but do not prepare separate meals for each. For example, one person shouldn't have much pungent taste, and if there's a pungent pickle, let's say, maybe that individual just tastes it, but doesn't have much of it. Someone else shouldn't have a very rich dessert so they have a few bites of the dessert. They just taste it and don't have very much. The point is that you don't cook a separate meal for each prakriti. There should be enough variety at each meal for everyone to select what is appealing and be satisfied. You simply need to understand the principles involved for each family member, and then it's very simple to serve balanced meals.

5.    **Question:** When can you drink milk and what should you not mix in milk?

**Answer:** It's best to drink milk by itself rather than as part of a meal. Actually, milk is sweet and that is why the sweet things can be added it. For example, a sweet fruit such as banana can be added to milk.

6.    **Question:** It's my understanding that Basmati rice is lighter than other rice, and can be eaten by Kapha types.

**Answer:** Basmati rice is good for Kapha in moderate amounts. All rice is included in a Kapha diet, but when we can choose one rice over others, we choose Basmati. Rice is a staple of the diet and can be eaten by everybody; only Kapha shouldn't take so much of it. And Kapha should fry the rice in a little ghee before boiling in water. Rice, wheat, and lentil dahls are perfect foods. They are the main grain foods which everyone can eat.

# *Questions and Answers about AyurVeda*

7.     **Question:** How do we get enough protein and follow a sattvic diet?

**Answer:** Many think that protein means only eating meat, including chicken, fish, or eggs. We advise avoiding animal flesh and eggs. Their effects are not good. They are not the only sources of protein. You can have a diet high enough in protein by eating dairy products, especially milk, as well as soups or dahls made from various lentils and served with rice. Black gram (urad lentils) have an abundant quantity of digestible protein.

8.     **Question:** I understand that we should eat foods that are fresh and grown locally. But lemons are not grown where I live, and yet they are something my AyurVedic doctor recommended that I have at each meal. What should I do?

**Answer:** By "local" we mean what our country grows. What is most suitable for us is what is grown in the United State.

9.     **Question:** Is it okay to eat hot foods like rice and dahl with cold foods, meaning cold temperature foods like salads, at the same meal?

**Answer:** Cold food is okay with rice and dahl. Salad is cool, not ice cold.

10.     **Question:** Is it all right to mix fruit and vegetables at the same meal?

**Answer:** According to AyurVeda, it is all right to eat fruit and vegetables in the same meal.

11.     **Question:** When food such as wheat is eaten in a dry form, like crackers, what influence will that have on the doshas?

**Answer:** Processing is an important point in AyurVeda. Wheat is heavy in quality. When made into crackers it becomes dry and light. Then it may be lighter to digest and better for Kapha types.

12.    **Question:** Should almonds be eaten with the skin on, or blanched to remove the skin, so that they're white?

**Answer:** It is better to remove the skin from the almond. Almond skin is sour in taste. Eating many unblanched almonds can give a little pain in the chest or heartburn. When we remove the skin, almonds add a sweet taste and are good for all doshas. Of course, in a large quantity even blanched almonds produce gas. But in moderation they are okay. Digestion of almonds is slow and heavy, so for Kapha small quantities are best.

13.    **Question:** Should I boil water for drinking?

**Answer:** Boiling water makes it lighter. Once or twice a day you might drink very warm water that has been boiled. This is a healthy habit to develop that is very good for digestion. But that doesn't mean that all day long we are to drink only warm water or we should never have any cool water. You may want to boil water and then cool it to room temperature to drink with meals and during the day.

14.    **Question:** I like pepper in soups but I heard Pitta-dominant people aren't supposed to eat it. What can I do?

**Answer:** The properties of black pepper are pungent, hot, light, dry, and rough. These properties promote digestion, increase Pitta and Vata, and decrease Kapha.    That doesn't mean if you are the body type that pepper increases, you should *never* have it. If black pepper is used excessively it will tend to exaggerate that particular dosha. If you're a Pitta type, black pepper certainly wouldn't be something you'd take in large quantities, especially in the summertime when Pitta is more predominant. And Vata types would avoid large amounts of black pepper in light and dry seasons.

15. **Question:** I have trouble waiting 3 to 6 hours before eating. Is it permissible to eat snacks between meals if I am hungry?

**Answer:** When you are hungry, you should eat. That is a rule of AyurVeda. But sometimes we are ruled by our own habits instead. That is not good. An occasional snack is not so bad. But always snacking will invite many types of digestive complications. If you eat to your satisfaction at mealtime, you won't have the habit of snacking.

16. **Question:** What is the best kind of milk to drink?

**Answer:** Although there are eight types of milk described in Ayur-Veda, cow's milk is the best. Goat's milk has a little lighter quality than cow's milk, and a little lighter to digest. But cow's milk is the most excellent for taste, appetite, and nutrition.

17. **Question:** Some people have this feeling that sugar isn't such a good thing to eat. Can sugar be eaten or should it never be eaten?

**Answer:** Eat either brown or white sugar in moderation. There is not some "magical" sugar from Vedic times. Because of its sweet, cold, heavy properties eating too much sugar aggravates Kapha dosha.

18. **Question:** What is the best way to drink milk?

**Answer:** It is best to heat milk before drinking. It shouldn't generally be taken right out of refrigerator and served. First, milk should be brought to a full boil, then cooled to a comfortably hot or warm temperature before drinking.

19. **Question:** I have heard some foods described as "auspicious." What does it mean?

**Answer:** A food that is especially life promoting, such as milk or ghee, is auspicious.

345

# 11  The AyurVeda Cookbook

# Appendices

Charts of Ingredients
Glossary
Sources
Index

# Charts of Ingredients

## Beverages

### Juices

| | VATA | PITTA | KAPHA | TASTE AND QUALITY |
|---|---|---|---|---|
| Apple | * | - | * | Sweet |
| Apricot | - | * | + | Sweet, Slightly Sour |
| Carrot | * | + | * | Sweet, Astringent, Hot |
| Cranberry | - | * | + | Sour, Sweet, Astringent |
| Coconut | * | * | + | Sweet, Oily, Heavy |
| Grapefruit | * | + | + | Sour, Sharp |
| Grape | * | - | + | Sweet, Cold |
| Lemon | - | + | + | Sour, Cold |
| Lime | - | - | + | Slightly Sour, Cold |
| Orange (sweet) | - | + | + | Sweet, Heavy, Hot |
| Orange (sour) | - | + | - | Sweet, Sour, Heavy |
| Papaya (ripe) | * | + | - | Sweet |
| Pear (ripe) | * | * | + | Sweet, Sour |
| Pineapple | - | - | + | Sweet |
| Pomegranate | - | - | * | Sweet, Astringent, Sour |
| Prune | - | - | + | Sweet, Sour, Heavy |
| Peach | - | - | + | Sweet, Slightly Sour |
| Tomato | - | + | + | Sour |

### Teas

| | VATA | PITTA | KAPHA | TASTE AND QUALITY |
|---|---|---|---|---|
| Chamomile | + | * | - | Bitter, Astringent |
| Peppermint | * | - | - | Pungent, Sweet, Sharp |
| Spearmint | * | - | - | Pungent, Sweet, Astringent, Sparkling, Sharp |
| Rosehips | - | + | * | Sour, Astringent aftertaste |
| Orange Pekoe (other black tea) | + | * | - | Astringent, Bitter |
| Jasmine | * | - | - | Astringent, Bitter, Sweet |

### Herbal Tea Blends

| | VATA | PITTA | KAPHA | TASTE AND QUALITY |
|---|---|---|---|---|
| Emperor's Choice | - | * | - | Sweet, Astringent, Bitter |

| | VATA | PITTA | KAPHA | TASTE AND QUALITY |
|---|---|---|---|---|

Increasing (+) or decreasing (-) or neutral effect (*)

# Appendices

| | VATA | PITTA | KAPHA | TASTE AND QUALITY |
|---|---|---|---|---|
| Mandarin Orange -Spice | - | * | - | Sour, Astringent |
| Raspberry | - | * | - | Sour, Astringent aftertaste |
| Red Zinger | | | | |
| (cold) | - | + | + | Slightly Sour |
| (hot) | - | + | - | Slightly Sour |
| Herbal Tea Blends | | | | |
| Pelican Punch | - | * | - | Sweet, Pungent, Astringent |
| Almond Sunset | - | + | + | Slightly Sweet, Bitter, Astringent |
| Cinnamon Rose | - | + | + | Slightly Sour, Astringent |
| Mocha Spice | + | * | - | Astringent, Bitter |
| Morning Thunder | + | * | - | Astringent, Bitter |
| Coffee | | | | |
| Decaffeinated | + | - | - | Bitter |
| With caffeine | + | - | - | Bitter |
| Iced Coffee | + | - | + | Bitter |
| **DAIRY PRODUCTS** | | | | |
| Milk (Cow's) | - | - | + | Sweet, Oily, Heavy, Cold |
| Skim milk | - | - | + | Sweet, Oily, Heavy, Cold |
| Cream | - | - | + | Sweet, Oily, Heavy, Cold |
| Buttermilk | - | + | + | Sour, Cold, Heavy |
| Butter | - | - | + | Sweet, Sour, Oily, Soft |
| Ghee | - | - | + | Sweet, Light, Cold |
| Sour cream | - | + | + | Sour, Cold, Heavy |
| Yogurt | - | + | + | Sour, Hot, Heavy, Oily |
| Cheese | | | | |
| Panir, Ricotta cheese | - | - | + | Slightly Sour, Oily, Cold |
| Cottage cheese | - | + | + | Sour, Cold |
| Semi-hard and Hard cheese | - | + | + | Sour, cold, heavy, oily |

| VATA | PITTA | KAPHA | TASTE AND QUALITY |
|---|---|---|---|

Increasing (+) or decreasing (-) or neutral effect (*)

# Charts of Ingredients

## HERBS AND SPICES

| | VATA | PITTA | KAPHA | TASTE AND QUALITY |
|---|---|---|---|---|
| Allspice | + | + | - | Pungent, Astringent |
| Anise | * | - | - | Sweet, Bitter, Astringent |
| Asfoetida | - | + | - | Astringent, Hot |
| Basil | - | + | - | Pungent |
| Bay Leaves | * | + | - | Bitter, Astringent |
| Caraway | - | * | + | Bitter, Astringent |
| Cardamom | * | - | + | Sweet, Bitter, Astringent, Hot |
| Cayenne | - | + | - | Pungent, Light , Dry |
| Celery seed | + | * | - | Pungent, Bitter |
| Chili pepper | * | + | - | Pungent , Dry, Hot |
| Cilantro | - | * | - | Pungent, Astringent, Bitter |
| Cinnamon | - | * | - | Pungent, Sweet |
| Cloves | - | + | - | Pungent, Hot, Light |
| Coriander | + | - | - | Sweet, Slightly Pungent, Oily |
| Cumin | - | + | - | Sweet, Bitter, Pungent, Light |
| Dill | - | - | * | Bitter, Astringent |
| Fennel | * | - | - | Sweet, Bitter, Astringent |
| Fenugreek | - | + | - | Sweet, Bitter, Hot |
| Garlic | - | + | + | Sour, Oily |
| Ginger | - | + | - | Pungent, Sweet, Light, Dry |
| Horseradish | + | + | - | Bitter, Light |
| Lemon thyme | * | + | - | Pungent |
| Licorice root | - | - | - | Sweet, Light |
| Mace | + | - | - | Bitter, Sweet, Dry |
| Marjoram | + | + | - | Pungent, Slightly astringent |
| Mustard | | | | |
| black seed | - | + | - | Pungent, Oily, Sharp, Hot |
| yellow seed | - | + | - | Pungent, Oily, Sharp, Hot |
| Nasturtium | - | + | - | Slightly Sweet, Pungent |
| Nutmeg | + | - | - | Bitter, Sweet, Dry |

Increasing (+) or decreasing (-) or neutral effect (*)

351

# *Appendices*

| | VATA | PITTA | KAPHA | TASTE AND QUALITY |
|---|---|---|---|---|
| Oregano | + | + | - | Pungent, Slightly Astringent |
| Paprika | + | * | - | Sweet, Slightly Pungent |
| Parsley | - | * | - | Pungent, Astringent, Slightly Bitter |
| Pepper-black | - | + | - | Pungent, Dry, Light, Hot |
| Poppy seed | - | * | + | Bitter |
| Rosemary | + | + | - | Astringent, Slightly Bitter, Sharp |
| Saffron | - | + | - | Sweet, Pungent,Smooth |
| Sage | + | + | - | Pungent, Astringent, Bitter |
| Salt | - | + | + | Salty, Smooth, Heavy |
| Savory | * | * | - | Pungent |
| Sesame Seed | - | + | + | Sweet, Astringent, Bitter |
| Tarragon | * | * | - | Pungent, Bitter |
| Thyme | + | + | - | Pungent,Astringent,Slightly Bitter |
| Turmeric | + | * | - | Bitter, Astringent, Hot, Dry |
| **CONDIMENTS** | | | | |
| Catsup | - | + | + | Sour, Sweet |
| Pickles- | | | | |
|   dill | - | + | - | Sour, Astringent |
|   sweet gherkin | - | * | - | Sweet, Slightly Astringent |
| Soy Sauce/ | | | | |
|   Tamari | - | + | + | Sour, Salty |
| Vinegar | + | + | - | Astringent, Light, Dry |
| Mustard | - | + | - | Pungent, Oily, Sharp |
| Black olives | - | + | + | Salty |
| Vanilla | * | * | * | Sweet |
| Chocolate | | | | |
|   semi-sweet | + | - | + | Bitter, Astringent, Sweet |
|   unsweetened | + | - | - | Bitter, Astringent |
| Honey | - | + | - | Sweet, Bitter, Astringent, Hot |
| Sugars | - | - | + | Sweet, Heavy, Cold |
| | **VATA** | **PITTA** | **KAPHA** | **TASTE AND QUALITY** |

Increasing (+) or decreasing (-) or neutral effect (*)

| | VATA | PITTA | KAPHA | TASTE AND QUALITY |
|---|---|---|---|---|
| Molasses | - | - | + | Sweet, Heavy |
| **LENTILS AND BEANS** | | | | |
| Mung and other Lentils | + | - | - | Astringent, Light, Dry, Cold |
| Urad lentils | - | - | + | Sweet, Astringent, Heavy, Oily, Hot |
| Other Beans | + | - | + | Astringent, Dry, Heavy |
| Tofu and other soybean products | * | - | + | Sweet, Heavy, Cold, |
| **NUT BUTTERS** | | | | |
| Peanut | - | + | + | Sweet, Sour, Heavy, Oily |
| Sesame | - | + | + | Sweet, Astringent, Oily |
| Raw Cashew | - | - | + | Sweet, Heavy, Oily |
| Almond (unblanched) | - | + | + | Sweet, Astringent, Hot, Oily Heavy |
| Almond (blanched) | - | - | + | Sweet, Heavy, Oily |
| Chocolate/ Macadamia | + | - | - | Sweet, Bitter, Astringent |
| **VEGETABLES** | | | | |
| Artichoke | - | - | + | Sweet, Heavy, Cold |
| Asparagus | - | * | + | Sweet, Oily, Heavy |
| Avocado | - | * | + | Sweet, Oily, Heavy |
| Bean sprouts | + | - | - | Sweet, Salty, Bitter, Light |
| Beets | - | - | + | Sweet, Astringent, Heavy |
| Beet greens | * | * | * | Sweet |
| Broccoli | + | - | - | Sweet, Astringent, Bitter, Dry |
| Brussel sprouts | + | - | - | Sweet, Salty, Bitter, Dry |
| Cabbage | + | - | - | Sweet, Salty, Bitter, Dry |
| Carrots | * | + | - | Sweet, Oily, Astringent, Hot |
| Cauliflower | + | - | * | Sweet, Salty, Astringent, Dry |
| Celery (raw) | + | - | - | Astringent, Dry, Light, Cold |
| Celery leaves | + | + | - | Bitter, Astringent, Pungent |

Increasing (+) or decreasing (-) or neutral effect (*)  353

# Appendices

| | VATA | PITTA | KAPHA | TASTE AND QUALITY |
|---|---|---|---|---|
| Celery(cooked) | - | - | + | Sweet |
| Cucumbers (peeled) | - | * | + | Sweet, Cold, Heavy |
| Eggplant | + | - | - | Sweet, Light, Dry |
| Green beans (well cooked) | - | * | - | Sweet |
| Lettuce | + | - | - | Sweet, Bitter, Pungent, Astringent, Light |
| Peas | + | * | - | Sweet, Astringent, Light |
| Peppers (sweet) | - | * | + | Sweet, Sharp |
| Peppers (hot) | * | + | - | Pungent, Astringent |
| Potato | + | - | + | Sweet, Astringent, Heavy, Dry |
| Radish | - | * | - | Pungent, Cold |
| Spinach | + | + | - | Astringent, Light, Hot, Dry |
| Tomato | - | + | + | Sweet, Sour, Light |
| Swiss chard | + | - | - | Bitter |
| Squash | + | - | - | Sweet, Dry, Heavy |
| Yam | * | - | + | Sweet, Astringent, Dry, Heavy |
| Zucchini | + | * | - | Bitter, Sweet, Cold |
| Zucchini (peeled) | * | * | - | Sweet, Astringent, Cold |
| **FRUITS** | | | | |
| Apples, green | - | + | - | Sour, Sweet, Light, Cold |
| Apples | + | - | * | Sweet, Astringent, Light, Cold |
| Apricots | - | * | + | Sweet, Slightly Sour |
| Banana | - | + | + | Sweet, Heavy, Smooth |
| Banana-chips (sweetened) | - | - | + | Sweet |
| Cherries (sweet) | - | - | + | Sweet, Heavy |
| Cherries (tart) | - | + | + | Sour, Heavy, Cold |
| Coconut | - | - | + | Sweet, Very Oily, Heavy |
| Cranberries | - | * | + | Sweet, Sour, Astringent |

|  | VATA | PITTA | KAPHA | TASTE AND QUALITY |

Increasing (+) or decreasing (-) or neutral effect (*)

# Charts of Ingredients

| | VATA | PITTA | KAPHA | TASTE AND QUALITY |
|---|---|---|---|---|
| Currants | - | - | + | Sweet |
| Dates | - | - | + | Sweet, Heavy |
| Figs (fresh/dried) | - | - | + | Sweet, Heavy |
| Grapes | - | - | + | Sweet, Cold |
| Grapefruit | - | + | + | Sour, Sharp |
| Kiwi | - | - | + | Sweet, Cold |
| Lemon | - | + | + | Sour |
| Lime | - | - | + | Slightly Sour |
| Mango | - | + | + | Sweet, Sour, Cold |
| Melons | - | - | + | Sweet, Cold, Heavy |
| Orange (sweet) | - | * | + | Sweet, Sour |
| Orange (sour) | - | + | + | Sour, Sharp, Heavy |
| Papaya | * | + | - | Sweet |
| Peaches | - | - | + | Sweet, Slightly Sour, Heavy |
| Pears, unripe | + | - | - | Sour, Slightly Sweet, Dry, Light |
| Pears (ripe or dried) | - | - | + | Sweet, Slightly Sour, Heavy, Cold |
| Persimmon | * | + | - | Sweet, Astringent |
| Pineapple (fresh) | - | - | + | Sweet Slightly Sour, Cold |
| Pineapple, (dried) | - | - | + | Sweet, Heavy |
| Pomegranate | + | - | - | Astringent, Sweet, Sour |
| Prunes/Plums | - | - | + | Sweet, Slightly Sour, Heavy |
| Raisins | - | - | + | Sweet |
| Raspberries | - | - | + | Sweet, Slightly Bitter |
| Strawberries | - | + | + | Sweet, Slightly Sour |
| Watermelon | - | - | * | Sweet, Light, Cold |
| **GRAINS** | | | | |
| Barley | + | * | - | Sweet, Astringent, Dry, Light |
| Corn | * | + | - | Sweet, Astringent, Hot, Light |
| Millet | * | * | - | Sweet, Light, Dry |

Increasing (+) or decreasing (-) or neutral effect (*)

# Appendices

| | VATA | PITTA | KAPHA | TASTE AND QUALITY |
|---|---|---|---|---|
| Oats | - | * | + | Sweet, Oily, Heavy |
| Rice brown & white- | | - | + | Sweet, Cold, Light, Oily |
| Rye | - | + | - | Sour, Hot |
| Wheat | - | - | + | Sweet, Cold, Oily, Heavy |
| **RICE CAKES** | | | | |
| Corn | - | + | - | Sweet, Light, Dry, Hot |
| Sesame | - | * | + | Sweet, Bitter, Astringent |
| 5 Grain | - | * | - | Sweet, Light, Dry |
| Barley & Oats | - | - | - | Sweet, Light, Dry, Little Oily |
| Sweet Rice | - | - | - | Sweet, Light |
| **OILS** | | | | |
| Coconut | - | - | + | Sweet, Very Heavy, Oily |
| Ghee | - | - | + | Sweet, Light, Cold, Oily |
| Olive oil | - | - | + | Sweet, Astringent, Oily |
| Sesame oil | - | + | + | Sweet, Bitter, Astringent, Oily |
| Sunflower/ Safflower oil | - | - | + | Sweet, Light, Oily |
| Margarine | - | + | + | Sweet, Astringent, Cold, Oily |
| **SEEDS AND NUTS** | | | | |
| Almonds (blanched) | - | - | * | Sweet, Heavy, Oily |
| Almonds (unblanched) | - | + | + | Sweet, Astringent, Hot, Oily |
| Pumpkin seeds (roasted) | - | - | * | Sweet, Astringent |
| Sesame seeds | - | + | + | Sweet, Bitter, Astringent |
| Sunflower (raw) | - | - | + | Sweet, Heavy |
| Sunflower (roasted) | - | - | * | Sweet, Light |
| Walnuts | + | - | - | Astringent, Bitter |
| Cashews | - | - | + | Sweet, Heavy |
| Peanuts | - | + | + | Sweet, Sour, Heavy |

Increasing (+) or decreasing (-) or neutral effect (*)

# Glossary

AGNI—(AHG-nee) Fiery, heating element in nature providing good digestive ability.

AMA—(AH-mah) Toxic substance resulting from improperly digested food, that passes "immaturely" through the digestive system and does not allow the plasma and body tissues to be formed on schedule. A source of many diseases.

APPETIZER—A good appetizer tastes pungent or warm, sweet, and unctuous or a combination of these. The colors red and gold are appetizing.

AUSPICIOUS FOOD—Food that is especially life promoting, in the superior or *sattvic* catagory.

AYURVEDA—(ah-yr-VAY-d) From the Sanskrit *Ayu* - life and *Ved* - knowledge. With a written history dating back more than 5,000 years, AyurVeda includes all aspects of life: consciousness, physiology, behavior, and environment.

DOSHAS—(DOH-shus) An imbalance in the physiology. According to AyurVeda, each person is naturally an identifiable constitutional type called Vata, Pitta, or Kapha, or sometimes a combination of two or all three. Vata is most like air and space, Pitta like water and fire, and Kapha earth and water. When these elements are out of balance they are called *doshas*.

GUNAS or food catagories—(*GOO-nahs*) The three catagories making up nature are, first, the pure, light, superior *sattva*; the second, active, energetic *rajas*, and third dull, sleepy *tamas*. All three gunas are found in living things.

KAPHA—(KAHF) A moist, cold, heavy, smooth, soft element.

MAHARISHI AYUR-VEDA—Maharishi Mahesh Yogi, founder of the Transcendental Meditation program, working closely with leading scholars and physicans, has restored the ancient science of AyurVeda to completeness.

PITTA—(PIT) Its properties are light, dry, hot, and energetic.

PRAKRITI—(PRAH-kri-tee) One's nature from birth, i.e., Vata, Pitta, Kapha, or a combination of these.

RASAYANAS—(rah-SY-uh-nahs) Foods that promote longevity. A rasayana contains all the nutrition needed for the development of every body tissue. "Rasa" denotes the first extraction in the digestive process that provides for the growth of the entire physical system

# Appendices

TRANSCENDENTAL MEDITATION (TM)--A simple mental technique, taught by Maharishi Mahesh Yogi, for gaining deep rest, happiness, improved health, and clear thinking. Especially useful in preparation for all activities including cooking. Recommended as a part of AyurVeda, Maharishi's TM program enhances all aspects of life.

VATA—(VAHT) From the Sanskrit *vayu*, it is most like air and space. Its elemental properties are dry, cold, windy, gaseous, and lightweight.

YAGYA—A special ceremony or gift with life-supporting and nourishing results for those involved.

## Sources

For Information and to order Maharishi Ayur-Veda Churnas, Teas, Rasayanas, and other products:

Maharishi Ayur-Veda Products International
P. O. Box 541
Lancaster, MA 01523
phone: 508-365-9643 or 1-800- All-VEDA
FAX: 508-368-7475

# Maharishi Ayurveda Medical Centers
# for
# North America

Maharishi Ayur-Veda Medical Center
National Office: United States
Box 282
Fairfield, Iowa 52556
515-472-8477

Maharishi Ayur-Veda Medical Center
Canadian National Office
190 Lees Avenue
Ottawa, Ontario K1S 5L5
613-235-0952

Austin: Maharishi Ayur-Veda Center
2 Sage Court
Austin, TX 78737
512-288-4309

Canada: Maharishi Ayur-Veda Medical Center
Box 6500
Huntsville, Ontario P 0A 1K0
705-635-2234

# *Appendices*

Detroit: Maharishi Ayur-Veda Medical Center
909 Woodward Avenue. Suite 117
Pontiac, MI 48053
313-858-8030

Houston: Maharishi Ayur-Veda Health Center
5508 Chaucer Street
Houston, TX 77005
713-526-6001

Los Angeles: Maharishi Ayur-Veda Medical Center
17308 Sunset Boulevard
Pacific Palisades, CA 90272
213-454-5531

Massachusetts: Maharishi Ayur-Veda Health Center
679 George Hill Road
Lancaster, MA 01523
617-365-4549

Boston: Maharishi Ayur-Veda Center
33 Garden St.
Cambridge, MA 02138
617-876- 4581

New York: Maharishi Ayur-Veda Center
45-05 Francis Lewis Boulevard
Bayside, New York 11361
5116-754-1466

Palm Beach: Maharishi Ayur-Veda Center
220 Sunrise Avenue
Palm Beach, FL 33480
407-832-4500

San Francisco: Maharishi Ayur-Veda Health and Education Resources
347 Delores St.
San Francisco, CA 94110
415-255-1928

St. Louis: Maharishi Ayur-Veda Center
Star Route #1 - Box 196
Ste. Genevieve, MO 62670
312-756-8011

Washington D.C.: Maharishi Ayur-Veda Medical Center
21112 F Street, NW
Washington, D.C. 20037
202-785-2700

International: Maharishi World Center for Ayur-Veda
Director of International Health Services
Maharishi Nagar
Noida, 201 307, India

To order copies of THE AYURVEDA COOKBOOK: COOKING FOR LIFE
by Linda Banchek or to arrange AyurVedic cooking talks, consultations, or
presentations contact:

Orchids & Herbs Press
503 W. Burlington
Fairfield, Iowa 52556
1-800-729-8803

# Appendices

# Index

Agni 7, 12, 14, 15, 16, 23, 43, 194, 196, 197
Almond Custard Fresh Fruit Pie 93, 299
Aluminium 137
Ama 15
American 3, 14, 67
  Apple Pie 179, 184, 300
  cooking. 94
  cuisine, 95
  food 181
  main dishes. 95
  Picnic Menu 179
Indian Menu 148
An Annual Fast 194
Appetite 6, 26, 48, 145, 197, 345
Appetizer 12, 23, 26, 43, 68, 159, 198
Apple Dumplings 301
Apple Pie Filling without Sugar 185, 303
Apple-Raisin Chutney 157, 244
Asparagus Salad in Raspberry Vinaigrette 30, 229
Attention 132, 145
Auspicious 345
Autumn 42, 91
Avocado Cheese Sauce and Dip 239
AyurVeda 3, 7, 8, 10, 14-17, 21, 89, 90, 93, 95, 132, 133, 145, 155, 194-198, 343, 345
AyurVedic
  cook 95, 131, 135
  Cooking 6, 89, 135, 96
  Food 3, 14
  Kitchen 131
  kitchen garden 133
  meal 131, 146
  menu 24, 44
  nutrition 6
Baby's Diet 198
Baked Lentil Soup 93, 203, 260
Baked Wild Rice Casserole 93, 271
Balance 4, 16, 17, 23, 24, 66, 67, 93, 94, 95, 139, 190
Balanced meals 8, 342
Barley 67, 68, 79, 201
Basic Pitta Broth 46

Basmati rice 200, 342
Bed and Breakfast Drink 217
Body building 23
Body types 5, 8, 89
Breakfast 14
Butter Pie Crust 184, 307
canned and frozen foods 136
Caraway Dressing 93
Carbonated drinks 17, 23, 200
Cashew Nut Balls 148, 164, 309
Categories of Diet 13, 90
Cereals 9, 10, 25
Charaka Samhita 11
Cheese Crackers 93, 172, 173, 224
Children 94, 210
Chocolate 9, 96
Chocolate Custard Pie 27, 34, 304
Chutneys and Other Condiments 148, 155
Clara Berno 196
Cleanliness 134
Climate 16, 17, 198
Coconut Chutney 158, 245
Coleslaw With Caraway Dressing 45, 49, 93, 230
Common sense 16, 18, 90, 197
Condiments 93, 94, 137, 139, 147, 155, 179
Confetti Rice Salad 179, 182, 231
Constitutional types 4, 5, 12
Cooking Methods 135
Cornbread 70, 75, 93, 255
Couscous 93, 280
Cream Tahini Sauce 241
Creamy Rice Pudding 27, 33, 329
Creamy Summer Garden Soup 45, 261
Curried Herb Cheese Dip 28, 93
Curried Squash Soup 204, 262
Curried Vegetables and Panir 93
Dahl 149
Deanna's Vinaigrette 241
Digestion 6-12, 15, 23, 26, 43, 156, 162, 197, 344
dosha 4, 12, 44, 65, 91, 92, 93, 192, 343
Dressings, Sauces, Marinades, Dips 237

English Cream 323
Enjoyment 6, 16, 17, 146
Environment 16, 23, 194, 198
Equipment and utensils 137
Fagioloni In Umido Volponi 172, 175
Fast Couscous 280
Fasting 15, 93, 193, 195
Flavored Cooking/Salad Oil 238
Food storage 136
Fragrantly Spiced Lassi 148,165, 217
French Bread 166, 170, 256
French Menu 166
French Potato Soup 93
Fresh Ginger Cookies 70, 75
Fresh Ginger Lemon Chutney 159, 226
Fresh Green Chutney 156, 245
Fresh Spinach Purée 204
Fried-Spiced Potatoes 152, 290
Fruit Shortcake 319
Ghee 91, 93, 96, 97, 197, 199, 201, 345
Ginger Carrot Soup 27, 29, 93, 263
Ginger Cookies 310
Ginger Soy Gravy 93, 242
Ginger Spice Cake 93, 320
Golden Yummies 69, 70, 96, 227
Good for all doshas 70, 159, 175, 183,
Green Beans in Tomato Sauce 175
Gunas 90
Hazelnut Cookies 90, 311
Health 3, 4, 7, 21, 65, 90, 190, 194, 202,
    344
Herbal Tea 93
Herbal Vinegar 237
Herbed Vinaigrette 238
honey 9, 17, 25, 54, 68, 79
How Ingredients Combine 95
Indian Spiced Milk Tea 218
Italian Menu 172
Italian Bread 93
Italian Hazelnut Cookies 172, 178
Jam Diagonals 312
Kaffa's Dream 330
Kapha 4, 6, 8, 10- 14, 18, 21, 24, 26, 34,
    48, 65- 69, 74, 89, 92,  96,138, 152, 154,
    159, 161-177, 180-184, 189, 203, 342-345

Kapha Broth 71, 254
Kapha Characteristics 65
Kapha dosha 150
Kapha types 95
Kapha's digestion, 68
Kapha-balancing 41, 65, 77
Kapha-increasing 13, 190
Kapha-Pitta 41, 92, 93
Kapha-Pitta-Vata 65
Kapha-reducing 67, 71, 75, 93, 150, 190
Kapha-reducing tea 190
Kapha-Vata 92
Kashmir 159
Kashmiri Mint Chutney 159, 246
Kaya Kalpa  196
Khichari 205, 264
Laddu 164, 309
Lassi 165
Leftovers 133
Lemon And Lime Wedges 162
Lemon Sauce 321
Lemon Scones 332
Lemony Date Bars 313
Light Food Fast 193
Liquid Fast 194
Light meals 14, 93, 193
Lightly Seasoned Vegetables 210, 277
Little Flat Breads 45, 48, 50, 257
Macedonia di Fruita 67, 172, 177, 232
Maharishi Ayur-Veda physicians 4,21,
    65, 189
Maharishi Ayur-Veda Program for
    Mothers and Babies. 196
Maharishi Mahesh Yogi 3, 90, 131, 143
Marble Crumb Cake 322
Marinate Tofu 47
Masoor Dahl 149, 265
Menu Planning 89, 93, 94
Menu Planning by the Season 91
Menu Planning for Kapha 66
Menu Planning For Pitta 42
Menu Planning for Vata 23
Microwave cookery 135
Milk 9, 11, 54, 66, 91, 96, 135, 193, 194,
    199, 341, 342, 343, 345

# Index

Moderation 345
Moroccan Delight 45, 47, 50, 278
Mother's Laddu 211, 314
New Mothers 196, 199, 208
Nursing 197
Nutrition 6, 7
Oatmeal Raisin Cookies 45, 51, 315
Oil Pastry 308
Old Fashioned Cake 93
Old Fashioned Tea Cake 93,324
One Full Meal Fast 193
Oven Baked French Fries 179, 181, 281
Panir and Ricotta Soft Cheese 250
Pasta And Green Sauce 172, 174, 281
Peas Braised with Lettuce 168, 282
Peche Cardinal 166, 171, 333
Petit Pois Braise Laitue 166, 168, 282
Pineapple Ginger-Cream Spread 28, 228
Pineapple Ice 45, 50, 334
Pineapple Mint Tea 219
Pitta 4, 6, 8-14, 18, 21, 24, 26, 34, 41, 43,
    48, 51, 52, 65, 66, 89, 92, 150-154, 157,
    159-165, 168, 170,171, 173, 176, 180-
    185, 189, 193, 197, 207-208, 344
Pitta Broth 253
Pitta Characteristics 41
Pitta Churna Dressing 49, 93, 235
Pitta constitution 43, 138
Pitta dosha 44, 160
Pitta Dressing, 93
Pitta-balancing 41, 42, 43, 52, 54, 93
Pitta-Kapha 41, 92, 93
Pitta-reducing 43, 45, 46, 49
Pitta-Vata 41, 92
Plain Refreshing Lassi 219
Pois Braise Laitue 168, 282
Potage Printanier/French Potato Soup
    166, 167, 266
prakriti 341, 342
Pressure Cooker 136
Puris 93
Puris and Chapatis 93, 148, 163, 258
Puris or Chapatis 148
Qualities 8, 10, 17, 44, 66, 89, 90, 94, 95,
    138, 190, 192, 342

Qualities for Vata 23
Questions and Answers about Ayur-
    Veda 341
Quick Coconut Condiment 162
Quick Vegetable Medley 206, 283
R&S Couscous 335
Raita 93, 148, 154
Rajas 91
Rasayana 90
Raspberry Vinaigrette 27, 30, 229
Recipe Design 94
Recipes For New Mothers 202
Refrigerator 136
Rice 91, 94, 137, 147, 197, 201, 251, 342,
    343
Rice Pilaf 168
Rich Quick Chocolate Mousse 336
Rich Stuffed Green Peppers 27, 31, 284
Roasted And Spiced Barley 70
Rose Petal Milkshake 220
saffron 8, 10, 25, 68, 96
Saffron Milk Tea 220
Saffron Rice 93, 292
Salt 4, 9, 25, 67, 80, 96, 194
Satisfaction 3, 14, 24, 145, 345
Sattvic 90,132, 343
Scrumptious Sesame-Orange Dressing
    and Sauce 243
Similarities and differences 6, 17, 91
Simple Cookie Crust 308
Simple Rice Pilaf 166, 169, 286
Simple Shortbread 212, 316
Simple Vinaigrette Dressing 74, 182, 231
Simply Baked Carrots 206, 285
Snacking 14, 15, 23, 68, 191, 345
Special Diets 189
Spiced Cashew Nuts 161, 247
Spiced Vegetable Curry 148, 150, 287
Spinach And Chicory Salad 172, 176,
    233
Splendid Layers Salad 45, 48, 234
spring 21, 43, 65, 92, 194
Squash Rolls 27, 33, 93, 259
Storing flours and Grains 137
Storing root crops 137

Strawberry Yogurt Pie 93, 305
Stuffed Artichokes with Herb Cheese 93
Stuffed Pasta Shells 93, 289
Sugar 9, 25, 42, 44, 67, 79, 96, 194,199, 201, 345
Summer 41, 43, 92, 341
Summer Garden Soup 45
Super Chocolate Brownies 179, 183, 317
Swedish Chocolate Cream Pie. 93, 306
Sweet Chocolate Cake With Cherry Sauce 325
Sweet Curry and Saffron Rice 148
Sweet Fruit and Spice Tea Bread 327
Sweet Fruit Smoothies 221
Sweet Potato-Apple Pie 207, 307
Sweet Potato Soup 208, 267
Sweet Summer Curry 152, 290
Tastes 4, 8, 13, 22, 44, 66, 67, 89, 90, 95, 138, 190, 192, 197, 201, 341, 345
Television 132, 144
The Upanishads 89, 144, 147
Three-in-One Samhita Supreme 222
Time 16, 144, 145, 192, 198
TM program 132
To Blanch Peppers 31
To Make Ghee 251
Tomato and Cucumber Raita 154
To Sprout Whole Beans and Seeds 72, 251
Toasted Coconut Condiment 153, 247
Toasty Cinnamon Bar Cookies 318
Tofu Nut Burgers 93,179, 180, 293
Tomato Chutney 160, 248
Tossed Green Salad 70, 74,93, 95, 166, 179, 236
Transcendental Meditation 132
Vanilla Sauce 302, 323
Variable Vegetable Soup 209
Vata Broth 30, 209, 252
Vata diet 34
Vata dosha 157
Vata menu 26
Vata-balancing 21, 23, 41, 93, 196, 198
Vata-Balancing Diet for New Mothers 201

Vata-Kapha 92, 93
Vata-Kapha, 21
Vata 4-8, 10-14, 18, 21, 23, 26, 34, 51, 65, 66, 89, 92, 96, 138, 150, 152, 159, 161, 162, 164, 168, 170-176, 180, 181, 182, 184, 185, 189, 193, 196, 198, 203, 207, 208, 213, 342, 344
Vata-Pitta 21, 41, 92
Vata-Pitta-Kapha 92
Vata-Pitta-Kapha 21
Vata-reducing 21, 26,210
Vegetable Barley Saute 69, 71
Vegetable Soup With Fresh Herbs 69, 71, 93, 268
Vegetable Whole Grain Sauté 296
Vegetables with Spiced and Roasted Barley 73, 294
Warm Water Fast 194
Water 192, 193, 194, 344
Watermelon Strawberry Punch 179,186
Weather 7, 16, 21, 41, 44, 65, 91, 92, 93
Weight loss 10, 15, 65, 75, 167, 189-191, 195, 196
White Figs in Apricot Cream Sauce 93, 337
White Figs A La Kapha 70, 76, 337
Winter 21, 43, 91, 341
Yagya 96, 131
Zucchini And Tomato Fry 27, 31, 93, 298

# Acknowledgement

I wish to thank all those who helped with this project, especially Dr. Haridas S. Kasture and Dr. Pramod D. Subhedar, leading experts in contemporary Ayur-Veda, for sharing their vast knowledge and helping me research AyurVeda and the American cuisine. I am particularly grateful to them for the many times they acted as cheerful subjects, in what can only be called food experiments, who tasted—in the name of Science—many unfamiliar western foods. My thanks, too, to the invaluable doctors and staff of the Maharishi Ayur-Veda Association of America in Fairfield, Iowa. To Joel Silver, M.D., who originated this book, Richard Averbach M.D., and Stuart Rothenberg, M.D., whose class "Ayurvedic Diet and Menu Planning" served as the basis for the text, and to the Department of Continuing Education at Maharishi International University for offering its unique series of courses in Maharishi Ayur-Vedic Science. And thanks to dear Clara Berno, good friend of hundreds of mothers and babies.

My thanks also to all the cooks and recipe developers for their contributions: Pamela Volponi, Tim and Lisa Messenger, Deanna Freeberg, Joanne Madden, Ulricke Selleck, Alan Scherr, Rick Weller, Jan Thatcher, Teresa Mottet, Bruce Rash, Judie Hickey, Lois Ducombs, and especially Elaine Arnold, who was always willing to make (and sample) just one more test-batch of brownies, and draw the pictures for the book, too. A special debt of gratitude goes to Ken Beaton; and to Pat Hurst, lover of good food, who tested and re-tested recipes, developed new ones at a moment's notice, and helped at every research session.

For their computer/technical assistance the invaluable Jessie Nichols, Murray Foster, Paul Sindar, and David Gendron have my deep appreciation. For clear words about publishing my thanks to Melanie Brown, Denise Denniston Gerace, and Bill Cates. Thanks to Claudia Petrick, precise of pen and cheerful, always. And Shepley Hansen for this book's cover.

A very special acknowledgement goes to Sushil and Anjali Mahaldar of Maharishi Ayur-Veda Products International as well as to Deepak Chopra, M.D., and the entire staff of Maharishi Ayur-Veda Health Center in Lancaster, Massachusetts, for their assistance in seeing this book to completion.

And most of all I want to thank Maharishi Mahesh Yogi for getting all of us together.

# A Traditiional Bessing After Eating

## *Annadahta*
## *Tataha Bhokda*
## *Pakarta*
## *Sukhi Bhava*

In gratitude to *Annadahta* who supplies the food.

Without the supplier there is nothing to eat.

And to *Tataha Bhokda* who eats the food.

Without the eater there is no eating.

And to *Pakarta,* the cook.

Without the cook there is no meal.

All three must do their part.

And when all three are one,

*Sukhi Bhava*

everyone is happy.

## *Jai Guru Dev*